THE CANCER CRISIS IN APPALACHIA

KENTUCKY STUDENTS TAKE ACTION

EDITED BY NATHAN L. VANDERFORD, LAUREN HUDSON, AND CHRIS PRICHARD

Copyright © 2020 by Nathan L. Vanderford

Published by Kentucky Publishing Services
An imprint of The University Press of Kentucky

Editorial and Sales Offices: The University Press of Kentucky
663 South Limestone, Lexington, Kentucky 40508-4008
www.kentuckypress.com

ISBN 978-1-950690-03-9 (paperback)
ISBN 978-1-950690-04-6 (pdf)
ISBN 978-1-950690-05-3 (epub)

This book is printed on acid-free paper meeting
the requirements of the American National Standard
for Permanence in Paper for Printed Library Materials.

Manufactured in the United States of America

Contents

High School Student Essays

Undergraduate Student Essays

Preface

THERE ARE OVER 1.7 million new cancer cases each year in the United States and over 600,000 cancer-related deaths.[1] Out of all the states in the nation, Kentucky has the most significant cancer problem; with over 26,000 new cases of cancer and more than 10,000 deaths each year, our beautiful commonwealth ranks first in the nation in overall cancer incidence and mortality rates.[2] That's bad, but what's worse is that our cancer problem is greatest in the fifty-four counties that make up the Appalachian region of Kentucky; both cancer incidence and mortality rates are significantly higher in Appalachian Kentucky compared to the non-Appalachian region of the state, which, again, is already number one in the United States.[3] There are many reasons for the high rates of cancer in Kentucky, including high smoking rates, poor diets, inadequate exercise, low socioeconomic levels, low education attainment, and limited access to healthcare.[4] These statistics and facts clearly highlight that cancer is a complicated menace to our country as a whole, and especially to our state.

Cancer statistics are clearly important to inform our broad understanding of the impact of the disease; but data, ranks, and facts hide the personal stories of how cancer affects the nation, Kentucky, and individuals. Behind each statistical data point is a person's life and a family's life that has been forever changed. Cancer patients endure many ranges of physical, emotional, and mental extremes and hardships. The turmoil of a cancer diagnosis and one's cancer journey can turn the patient, their family, and often whole communities upside down and inside out.

I know this personally. On June 20, 2010 (Father's Day), my dad died very suddenly—within minutes—from a massive hemorrhage that was the result of lung cancer. He suddenly started coughing up blood in the basement of my childhood home, and by the time he walked up the basement steps, he collapsed and bled to death.

My dad was a heavy smoker for more than forty years, a Marine veteran who was heavily exposed to Agent Orange in the jungles of Vietnam, and a factory worker for many, many years. At work, he was exposed to fumes and industrial material containing deadly chemicals. Of all these factors, I believe it was his smoking that affected his physical health most negatively.

His smoking affected me as well. I remember as a kid getting sick and hating the smell of cigarette smoke in the house because it would make me even sicker, so I would hide my dad's cigarettes and lighter, which would make him very angry. Eventually, I would give his pack of Winston's back to him, and he would go on with his smoking. My cries for him to stop smoking were just not enough for him to beat the powerful addiction.

A few months after my dad's death, my mom was diagnosed with breast cancer. Luckily, her cancer was found early as the result of her standard, regularly scheduled mammograms, and she was treated successfully. Today, she is happy and healthy.

My personal experiences with cancer highlight two important aspects of cancer care: cancer prevention and early detection. On the prevention side, if we limit our exposure to such cancer risk factors as tobacco, our likelihood of developing cancer can drop significantly. On the early detection side, regular cancer screenings are critical for finding early signs of cancer that may be developing. When found early, cancer can sometimes be more easily and successfully treated.

My story highlights exactly what the essays in this book are about: the personal impact that cancer has on us all, how we view the causes of the disease, and what we think can be done to lower its prevalence.

The essays you are about to read were written by a group of twenty high school and five undergraduate students, all residents of Kentucky's Appalachian region, who are participants in the University of Kentucky Markey Cancer Center's Appalachian Career Training in Oncology (ACTION) Program. ACTION aims to train the next generation of oncology professionals who will help battle the cancer problem in Kentucky and beyond, and to increase knowledge among the citizens of the region about cancer, cancer disparities, risk factors, and behaviors that can be modified to lower one's risk of developing the disease.

These students have lived in Appalachia their entire lives and have seen how cancer affects their families, their friends, and their communities. The students have learned about the biology and epidemiology of cancer as part of the ACTION Program, which has allowed them to form their understanding of why cancer rates are so high in their communities.

For the essays, I gave the students a simple, nondescript prompt. I told them to write an essay of about two thousand words that would briefly introduce themselves; describe their personal experience with cancer; explain why they think cancer impacts Kentucky so harshly; and discuss what they think can be done to address Kentucky's cancer epidemic.

The students submitted their essays; they peer-reviewed and peer-edited them; and we—the editors—reviewed and edited them. Through the review and editing process, we worked together diligently to hone the stories, the writing, and the tone and to cite and reference facts and quotes while also balancing students' personal opinions and maintaining each students' voice.

So what is the purpose of these essays? Before getting to the purpose, let me tell you the origin of the idea of having the students write the essays. As part of the application process for ACTION, applicants wrote a short essay that described why they were interested in the program. For the high school component of ACTION, we received ninety-one applications for twenty open positions. I read each applicant's essay and was blown away by the compelling stories of their personal experiences with cancer. It was these very individual and raw stories that inspired this project.

Now, the purpose of the project. Nelson Mandela said, "Education is the most powerful weapon which you can use to change the world," and it is my ultimate hope that these essays will educate readers about cancer, cancer disparities, cancer risk factors, and modifiable behaviors. I hope some readers will change behaviors that could be putting them at risk for developing cancer. Perhaps someone will be inspired to stop using tobacco products. I hope some readers will get an overdue screening or seek care for a nagging pain. Perhaps readers will be inspired to help cancer patients and their families in some way or to create community events around cancer education or cancer prevention initiatives. Ultimately, through education, inspiration, and encouragement, I hope these essays will be an impetus for change that can aid in reducing some of the burden of cancer in Kentucky.

If current or former cancer patients read the book, I hope you find the essays encouraging and uplifting. These students have big hearts, smart minds, and a passion for understanding cancer in general and the personal battles each patient wages with the disease. Through this knowledge, these students are motivated to address cancer's burden so that fewer people will be impacted by the disease.

This project also allowed our students to dig deeper into cancer, its causes, and ways to address the disease in the population. Through this, I hoped that students would become more equipped in their overall understanding of cancer and more inspired to pursue a cancer-related career. After observing their growth in the summer of 2019, I strongly believe that this has happened. I think that if you asked any of the students, they would give you a laundry list of things they have learned as the result of writing and editing their essays and working with their counterparts in the peer-review and editing process.

In starting this project, specifically for the high school students, I did not anticipate that they would learn so much about composing and editing a written work. I initially took for granted the level of writing, storytelling, and research skills these students brought to the ACTION Program. I also did not foresee the variability in these skills between students. Through this project, I believe the students have strengthened their skills, and this will help them as they finish high school, go on to college, and pursue their professional dreams.

The essays are authentic and, in some cases, a bit raw. As you read the essays, keep in mind that the majority of them were written by high school sophomores and juniors. I am not sure about you, but I could not have written an essay like what you will read here as a high school sophomore or junior. In fact, I probably still couldn't write such a story to this day.

I am extremely proud of the students' work; they have worked very, very hard on these essays, putting in many hours in the initial writing stage, the review stage, and the revision stage. I am proud of the stories told. I am proud of all that the students have learned through this process. I am proud of the impact the students will have on their families and communities through this project.

Like the students, I have also learned a lot through this project. Most importantly, I am more convinced than ever that the future of Kentucky, and our nation, is in great hands. The students have the drive, the energy, and the intellect to do remarkable things, including making a significant impact on the burden of cancer in Kentucky and beyond.

As you read through this book, I think you will be compelled by the students' personal stories of their experiences with cancer and their ideas, and I believe you will be inspired by the promise these students hold. I also believe you will be prompted to consider ways to take better care of yourself, your family, and your community.

I hope you enjoy this collection of essays.

Nathan L. Vanderford, PhD, MBA
Director, Appalachian Career Training
in Oncology (ACTION) Program

Notes

1. CDC/National Center for Health Statistics, "Leading Causes of Death," 2016, retrieved from https://www.cdc.gov/nchs/fastats/leading-causes-of-death.htm. R. L. Siegel, K. D. Miller, and A. Jemal, "Cancer Statistics, 2019," *CA Cancer J Clin* 69 (2019): 7–34, retrieved from https://onlinelibrary.wiley.com/doi/epdf/10.3322/caac.21551.

2. American Cancer Society, "Cancer Statistics Center: Kentucky," 2019, retrieved from https://cancerstatisticscenter.cancer.org/#!/state/Kentucky. Siegel, "Cancer Statistics."

3. Health Disparities 2017, "Creating a Culture of Health in Appalachia: Disparities and Bright Spots," 2017, retrieved from https://www.arc.gov/images/appregion/fact_sheets/HealthDisparities2017/KYHealthDisparitiesKeyFindings8–17.pdf. S. D. Rodriguez, N. L. Vanderford, B. Huang, and R. C. Vanderpool, "A Social-Ecological Review of Cancer Disparities in Kentucky," *South Med J* 111 (2018): 213–19.

4. M. Charlton, J. Schlichting, C. Chioreso, M. Ward, and P. Vikas, "Challenges of Rural Cancer Care in the United States," *Oncology (Williston Park)* 29 (2015): 633–40. Health Disparities 2017. A. M. Lopez, L. Hudson, N. L. Vanderford, R. Vanderpool, J. Griggs, and M. Schonberg, "Epidemiology and Implementation of Cancer Prevention in Disparate Populations and Settings," *ASCO Educational Book* 39 (2019): 50–60. Rodriguez, "Social-Ecological Review of Cancer Disparities." S. Zuppello, "The Cancer Capital of America," *The Outline*, 2019, retrieved from https://theoutline.com/post/7457/the-cancer-capital-of-america?zd=1&zi=qvjmrf2u.

HIGH SCHOOL STUDENT ESSAYS

Cancer
The Emotional Side

William Adams

WHAT DOES IT mean to have an interest in the medical field? If you had asked me this question five years ago, I would not have been able to give you an answer that you could have relied on. Five years ago, my heart was set on pursuing a business career and becoming a real estate agent. But roughly two years ago, I found out that my great-great-grandpa, Dr. Benjamin Franklin Wright, was a doctor of internal medicine. Another intriguing fact that I found was that Dr. Wright had helped many people in a fatal train accident in 1917. He was the only doctor in the town at the time who had enough skill to treat everyone who had gotten hurt. The only skill he lacked was surgical training. This would later cause him to reenter medical school, becoming a first-rate surgeon. This got me thinking: if he could do that, imagine what I could do. I was asking around my town for someone to guide me, and my pediatrician at the time suggested family medicine. This got me to thinking about being a family physician and made me fall in love with the idea. Ever since then I have been obsessing over the intriguing job of family physician. Me being nosey and pushy, I would ask doctors what they knew, and I would constantly Google random facts, such as, "How many clinical injuries does a family physician receive per year?" or "How many jobs are open to family physicians at the moment?" One night, I was scrolling through Google, trying to educate myself on all medical related subjects, and I saw an advertisement from a hospital that was in critical need of oncologists. An oncologist is a medical practitioner qualified to diagnose and treat tumors. I was interested and clicked the link, and it took me to a page of everything about oncology. I quickly read up on the position and was very intrigued. Over the next couple of days, I was reading and asking questions, and then I stumbled across the fascinating job of pharmaceutical oncologist, which is the main person who focuses on drugs to fight off the cancer. Somewhat shocked that I had finally found something that I liked and that suited my needs, I made that my top priority. My name is William Adams, and this is my journey with all things oncology.

I currently reside in the small county of Letcher. With a population of 23,000 and a 339-square-mile size, we are, you could say, a small town. If the numbers do not persuade you, maybe the fact that everyone was in uproar about finally getting a Taco Bell will. With the perks of living the small country life, such as knowing everyone and people being very nice, come the cons. When you live in a small town, you start to see that everyone knows one another. It starts off as going to a local place and greeting almost everyone. Then you find yourself hearing awful news. You hear that many have contracted a variety of diseases, one being cancer. When someone tells you that someone has contracted cancer, you cannot help but feel sympathy for that person. Being told you or someone else has cancer is something I would never bestow on someone.

This leads to an experience that I had with learning that someone close to me was affected by cancer. I found out that my great-uncle had contracted prostate cancer. As a child, and even right now, I have never really been close with him. This means that the news, even though he is part of my family, was not as harsh to me. The real struggle came when I found out my grandpa also had contracted prostate cancer. This was heartbreaking to my family and especially me, mainly because my grandpa was my best friend. Prostate cancer mainly affects the lower part of the body and can cause physical impairment. My grandpa would often have leg pain and back pain and trouble walking, and he would often have to take Flomax to get his kidneys active and running properly. He also used a catheter throughout his battle with prostate cancer, because it affected his urinary system. My grandpa had to take thirty-seven treatments of radiation to clear his prostate cancer, and this treatment did not come without a price. His battle with prostate cancer affected not only him but also the people closest to him. As I said before, my grandpa was my best friend, meaning we did many things together. I, being around eight years old, was always clueless about what was going on around me. I remember always wondering why he would take off for long periods of camping and hunting with me, and why he would be active on some days and not active on others. This would have me and my family discouraged and sad. Now that I am older and more mature, I finally understand that my grandpa had bigger things to deal with in his life.

Although my family has had a hard time dealing with cancer, we are not the only family that has. Many people in Kentucky have been diagnosed with many forms of cancer, some being very invasive, aggressive, and deadly. Kentucky has the highest rate of cancer in all of America. In my opinion, the fault should go to the population. Kentucky is known for having the highest rate of tobacco use, obesity, drug usage, and poverty in all of America. The most common form of cancer in Kentucky is lung cancer. This is mainly caused by smoking tobacco products. Lung cancer also causes the most deaths in Kentucky related to cancer. That is, lung cancer often lies dormant until it spreads throughout the body and eventually becomes untreatable and results in death most of the time.[1]

With the spike in lung cancer, another cancer-causing factor is making its way up the line: obesity. With the rise in unhealthy fast food joints, and the decline in work motivation, as well as low physical exercise, obesity rates have never been higher. Obesity cannot cause cancer directly, but it does leave you vulnerable to many types. Obese people often have chronic inflammation, which can lead to DNA damage and then cancer. Fat tissue also produces excess amounts of estrogen, which can lead to endometrial, breast, ovarian, and other cancers.

I also personally think that drug usage plays a bigger role in cancer than what most people think. Even though illicit drug usage cannot cause cancer directly, it does not mean users are in the clear. Methamphetamine, the most abused drug in Kentucky, can leave you the most vulnerable. Many forms of methamphetamine contain the substance benzene in it, which is a carcinogen. Individuals also engage in polydrug abuse, commonly known as "sharing needles." This can leave you prone to many health issues, ones that can compromise your immune system and make you vulnerable to many cancers. This information makes you realize the overall damage drugs can do to your body and why drugs are not the best choice for your health.

In Kentucky, many people live in poverty. Over half of Kentucky's population makes under $30,000 a year, which means they cannot afford many health-related opportunities. Being poor is a greater health threat than many people realize. When people live in poverty, they usually do not have access to health insurance, and that leaves them unable to get cancer screenings. Not getting a cancer screening can leave you clueless until it becomes too late and untreatable. Poverty can also cause many health concerns. If you are living close to other residents (through co-housing or in homeless situations), you are at risk of contracting many diseases that can leave you vulnerable to many cancers.

As I was writing this, my grandma told me a story about why she thinks Kentuckians have such a high rate of cancer. She told me that she was told about how people had dumped a large amount of chemicals into abandoned coal mines. Eventually, the chemicals had seeped through the mines and into the streams and lakes. The seeping left many humans exposed to these harsh chemicals. This would make logical sense considering how harsh humans are to their environment.

Kentuckians could never eradicate cancer—that is the cold, hard truth of it all. As a state, there are measures we could possibly take to lower the cancer incidence and death rates. One major step is to quit tobacco use. Kentucky's death rate for lung cancer is 66 per 100,000, not like the usual 42.[2] In my opinion, the best way to lower the tobacco-related cases is to raise the age to buy tobacco products. Taking into consideration that we cannot eradicate smoking entirely, raising the buying age would be the next best step. Obesity can also be treated. The biggest problem for low-income people is that junk food costs are lower than those of healthy foods. Kentucky should lower the healthy food prices and raise the junk food prices. I feel that that would make a big difference in how we eat our meals. We could also lower the number of fast food restaurants and check what they are serving to keep it within reasonable health standards and safety. Drug usage is a lot like tobacco use, addictive and uncontrollable. I feel that if we could eradicate drug abuse as a whole, we would gain a big step toward lowering the cancer rate. We should be strict on drug charges and eliminate gateway drugs such as marijuana. Poverty is the hardest problem to solve, as this is a countrywide issue. In my opinion, the reason why many people live in poverty is because prices are going up, but income is not. This leaves many people struggling to buy the necessities, such as insurance or often doctor visits, not to mention food and other necessities. If the government would raise income and lower prices, then many people would be able to afford insurance and could get cancer screenings. Many of these things apply not just to Kentucky but also to America as a whole. If something drastic is not done, cancer rates will keep rising and become an epidemic that we may never be able to control.

Imagine living a happy life. You have a nice job, house, and great kids. You think nothing in this world could possibly get you down. Then you go to the doctor for a simple checkup, and you get told the most disturbing news. You have cancer. What would you do? There is not a set answer on the things you could do. You actually could not do much because cancer defines your fate for you. A major thing you could do now is ease the risk of contracting cancer in the first place. You can do this by not using tobacco products, by eating healthier, and by getting educated in general and specifically about cancer. If you or someone you know can follow these difficult steps, you could possibly save your life and give ease to the loved ones around you. You are the only one standing in front of you and preventing you from seeing your loved ones again, so make the right decisions when it comes to your health and safety.

I might be from Letcher County, the smallest of all counties, and I might not be a specialist about cancer, but take advice from someone with personal experience. Losing someone to cancer is not fun, and it will never be. You can ask anyone who has ever lost someone to cancer—it is not an experience that anyone should have to go through. Be the change for yourself, your loved ones, and America itself. Do not end up a cancer casualty because you did not listen to valuable advice.

Notes

1. S. Becker, *Cancer in the U.S.: 15 States With the Highest Rates of Cancer Diagnoses,* June 19, 2018, retrieved from Cheat Sheet, https://www.cheatsheet.com/culture/cancer-in-the-us-states-with-the-highest-rates-of-diagnoses.html/. C. Blackburn, *Cancer Kills Kentuckians at Highest Rate (Update),* March 28, 2016, retrieved from North American Association of Central Cancer Registries, https://www.naaccr.org/cancer-kills-kentuckians-at-highest-rate/. L. Cahn, *The 20 States with the Highest Cancer Rates,* October 22, 2019, retrieved from The Healthy: https://www.thehealthy.com/cancer/states-with-the-highest-cancer-rates/.

2. Becker, *Cancer in the U.S.*

Cancer in Eastern Kentucky

Natalie Barker

KENTUCKY, MY HOME, is affected by cancer more than any other area in the United States. According to the Centers for Disease Control and Prevention (CDC), we have the highest incidence and mortality rates in the country.[1] This is not just a statistic to the citizens in Kentucky. What we are experiencing is a true crisis. Our community has been affected by cancer in unimaginably horrible ways. There is not a single person I know who has grown up and not been affected by cancer in some way. It is such a common occurrence in my community that people often treat the news of someone they know being diagnosed with cancer as just a common event.

I am a student from Elliott County, Kentucky, a rural area with so few people it doesn't even have a stoplight. Once I graduate high school, I plan on seeking higher education and pursuing a career in the medical field. Since I come from such an impoverished town, following this path will prove to be a challenge. Although it will be difficult, I plan on pushing through and following my dream of working in a field where I can directly assist my own community. Ever since I was first asked what I wanted to be when I grew up, I knew I wanted to help the people in my community and others like mine who are suffering. I have decided the medical field is the path I want to take due to my love of science and my volunteering experience in our local nursing home and rehabilitation center. Specifically, I want to help the fight against cancer in my area. In March 2019, I was accepted into the Appalachian Career Training in Oncology (ACTION) Program. This program will assist me in reaching new heights in my career path that I cannot reach on my own. The experience the ACTION Program provides me will help me assist my own struggling community for years to come.

Similar to most of the residents of Eastern Kentucky, I have had many experiences with cancer. The first experience took place before I was even born, yet it played a large part in shaping my childhood. My great-grandfather's life was taken by lung cancer. Although I was not born early enough to meet him, I was always told numerous stories about him. I was told about his time serving in World War II and how proud my family was of him. My great-grandmother told me about how he would whistle, mocking the sound a bobwhite bird would make, and the birds would gather in the front yard. I always tried to do this when I was younger; it made me feel as if he hadn't really been stolen from our family by this horrible disease. I was comforted by loving stories about him before he was taken from my family. He gave just as much love as he received. When he passed, he left a hole in my family members' hearts, one I could see and understand even as a child. Things he left behind like old tools or things he had made remained untouched, just as he left them, for years. He was taken too soon by cancer. His story is just one of the millions of examples of the enormous heartbreak cancer has left behind in our area.

The next experience I had with cancer took place when I was in the first grade; my stepbrother was diagnosed with leukemia. Being so young, I did not know how to help him or handle this news. So I did what any little sister would do; I annoyed him to no end, like normal. I used to beg to play on his laptop or put lip gloss on him, pester him for piggyback rides, and follow him around everywhere he went. For a long time, this was my routine. He put up with it all with a smile too. He used to pick me up and hold me above his head, which was terrifying at the time to me since, in my head, he was "a million feet tall." I put my bows in his hair, possibly against his will, and I remember it being the funniest thing I had ever seen. He let me watch him play video games, and I'd cover my eyes before he shot someone on them. I only wish I would have covered my eyes for the truly scary things I would witness later on.

Soon, he was too weak for piggyback rides and could hardly pick me up anymore. I could no longer fix his hair and giggle about how funny it looked because all of his hair had fallen out. He stopped chasing me around the house and instead spent his days sleeping. I watched him break down in front of his dad because his best friend who was fighting cancer alongside him had died. He stopped joking around and laughing with me and, instead, worried about the fact he could die too. All I could do was watch as this person I looked up to just broke down under the pressure of this disease. I wish someone would have told me to cover my eyes through that.

The most recent experience I have had with cancer happened just last year. I began volunteering at my local nursing home, and being there opened my eyes to the vast number of people in my area who have cancer. I made friends with many of the residents, as I was there almost every week. My main job was to make sure that all the residents had ice water. Surprisingly, it was harder than it sounds. Each resident had a different way they wanted their cups: with no ice, with ice, half full, three-quarters full with only one ice cube, the list went on. I learned how everyone liked their cup and had the routine almost perfect. I say almost because one woman was just *never* happy with how I filled her water cup. She yelled at me to no end, and no matter what I did she always had me come back. I was always frustrated with this woman until one day, a day I will never forget, I sat her cup down, told her it was "the best I can do," then asked her how she was doing as I always did. She looked at me with a hateful expression, then it seemed to melt into a sad one. She told me one simple thing that made my heart break: "You're the only person that has talked to me all day."

I began to realize why she was never satisfied with that cup. She sat alone in her room all day. She had no family or friends who still visited her. Her room was empty and grey, and the only sound was the beeping of the machines in the room. She was not a person filled with contempt for the world as I had thought. She was just lonely. And as I prepared her cup over and over, I spoke with her about my day, and she griped about hers. She just wanted someone to talk with. After that day, I saved her cup for last every time, so I had plenty of time to talk to her. I came into her room, filled her cup, and sat down to talk for as long as I could. She never complained about the cup again, and we became friends. She told me about her life, all the adventures she had been on, and gossiped about whatever came to her mind. She seemed delighted when I came to visit; it made me feel that I was truly making a difference.

As time went on, I visited the nursing home less and less. I was simply too busy to volunteer every week. After about a month of not going, I went back to volunteer for the day. When I went into her room, there was a new resident staying there. I knew what had happened and didn't want to believe it. I went to a woman I knew, who was there every day to visit her mother. I asked her what happened and received news I never wanted to hear. She had passed away; she died of cancer. She died alone. Cancer took yet another innocent life and will never give it back.

These stories are not anything out of the ordinary for people here. Most people's lives have been altered by cancer much worse than mine. As mentioned above, Kentucky has the highest cancer incidence and mortality rates among men and women in the United States. [2]It is not just a statistic or a number here; it is real and terrifying. Cancer is taking our friends, our brothers and sisters, our parents and grandparents, our entire community. It is taking our loved ones and leaving nothing but heartbreak and sadness behind.

The culture of Eastern Kentucky heavily contributes to the crisis we are experiencing. Factors such as substance abuse and lack of adequate information are all contributing to our high rates of cancer incidence.

Substance abuse is a prevalent thing in Eastern Kentucky, especially tobacco use. My hometown has accepted this unimaginably horrible carcinogen into our society with open arms. It has gotten to the point at which the town holds a yearly festival called "The Tobacco Festival." According to the CDC, smoking tobacco is linked to 80–90 percent of lung cancer deaths in the United States. Along with this, the CDC has stated that half of the children exposed to secondhand smoke end up dying from lung cancer.[3] If residents of Eastern Kentucky knew that tobacco smoking is actually killing their community and children, they would not accept this part of their culture as happily as they do.

This leads to the next big issue in Eastern Kentucky related to cancer: inadequate education. Until I joined the ACTION Program, I knew very little about cancer and how to prevent it. Now, I have noticed that residents of my town are constantly putting themselves at risk of developing cancer at an alarming rate. The main risk factors I see residents in my area expose themselves to include alcohol abuse, poor diet, obesity, exposure to UV rays, and tobacco use. According to the National Cancer Institute, all of these factors are linked to developing cancer.[4]

The most reliable way to survive cancer is to protect yourself from getting it in the first place. Educating yourself and others is the best way to start. Cancer education programs should be implemented in Eastern Kentucky to help improve cancer literacy in the area. If residents know how to protect themselves, they have a chance of winning the war against this disease.

Eastern Kentucky is in a crisis. We have the highest cancer incidence and cancer mortality rates in the country. We are not just a scary statistic. We are people, human beings just like you. We go to school. We eat dinner with our families. We have birthday parties and barbeques just like everyone else, yet our loved ones are being taken from us. We are in desperate need of help, not only from outside assistance but from inside our community as well. Ending the struggle our community faces must start with each individual. Protect yourself from carcinogens, educate yourself, be sure to get screenings and tests when necessary, and do not be afraid to go to your doctor if you have any concerns. Be sure that your family and friends do these things as well. Each person has their own opportunity to fight in the war against cancer. Will you?

Notes

1. CDC, "United States Cancer Statistics," retrieved from https://gis.cdc.gov/Cancer/USCS/DataViz.html.

2. Ibid.

3. CDC, "What Are the Risk Factors for Lung Cancer?" n.d., retrieved from https://www.cdc.gov/cancer/lung/basic_info/risk_factors.htm.

4. NCI, "Risk Factors for Cancer," retrieved from: https://www.cancer.gov/about-cancer/causes-prevention/risk.

On the Breaking Point

Rachel Collins

ONE OF MY favorite quotes is by George Moore: "A man travels the world over in search of what he needs and returns home to find it." This is a constant reminder that no matter where I go or how far I go, I will always return home to these Kentucky mountains.

My name is Rachel Lena Collins. I am sixteen years old and a sophomore student at Clay County High School. I come from Manchester, a small town in southeastern Kentucky, which is, as *The New York Times* once said of this area, "the hardest place to live in the United States. Statistically speaking."[1] Despite this statement, I am still exuberant that I can say Manchester forever holds the key to my heart. I grew up the youngest of four children that my mother partly raised on her own. My mother, Ana Maria Collins (Tejeda-Nápoles), is a naturalized American citizen. She was born in Havana, Cuba, in 1964 and comes from a long line of Cuban military soldiers, going back to our ancestors from Imperial Spain. My maternal great-grandfather was José Miguel Nápoles, former commander and chief of the Cuban Army Corps of Engineers during the Batista regime. One of my distant maternal family members is José Ángel "Mantequilla" Nápoles, a famous boxer and former World Welterweight Champion. He is a long-lost cousin of mine. I grew up not knowing very much about my mother's side of the family, due to their unexpected and immediate departure from the grips of communist Cuba. When my mom came to the United States in October 1970 as a bright-eyed six-year-old, she moved to Los Angeles, California, with her mother and stepfather, where she was raised and lived for the next twenty-eight years.

My father was born at Red Bird Mission in Beverly, Kentucky, and is the eldest of three children. My mom met my father when she moved temporarily to Ft. Stewart, Georgia, in 1998. They married in 1999 and moved together to his hometown of Manchester, Kentucky, in 2001 after he left the U.S. Army and joined the Army National Guard. His maternal grandfather, my paternal great-grandfather, Oather Smith, worked in the coal-mining industry for thirty-two years. Back in the day, the coal industry was booming and made the family financially stable. However, it wasn't long after that he developed black lung (pneumoconiosis caused by inhalation of coal dust), and he was forced to retire due to his failing health. This caused a great amount of distress for everyone to see such a strong man succumb to the voracious disease.

My mother found it hard to find steady work in this small town, so she continued her studies and conducted her trainee volunteer hours to become a nationally certified EMT-Basic. During the weekdays, I watched my mom and her coworkers practice life-saving techniques, like blood draws, IV administration, and CPR. This is where I learned that it's not like the movies and that only about 15 percent of people are ever "brought back" using the CPR method. But despite this statistic, you never quit trying. You transfer the process to a higher level of care when you get to the hospital because that 15 percent isn't just a number, it's a person who should be given another chance to kiss their kids goodnight, go to work to support their family, or celebrate a birthday with friends and family. That 15 percent represents important lives too. As I grew up watching these things, I gained a strong interest and desire to help others. I cannot imagine my life without the possibility of giving back to this beloved community.

My teachers always asked me the same question: "Rachel, what do you want to be when you grow up?" My response has always been the same: "When I grow up, I would like to be a doctor or work in the medical field." As a child, it never occurred to me how much care, thought, and dedication it actually takes to be in the medical field. I grew up observing all the techniques my mom had to learn and practice to become proficient in saving lives. It was exciting at times, but definitely risky and frightening. I would like to pursue a career in which I know I can make a change in my community or in other places of the world. I would be satisfied to have the opportunity to serve others with the latest information and techniques that could potentially heal the lives of many, even if just one at a time. Everyone is ultimately important, and their lives hold inestimable value.

Unfortunately, cancer has been no stranger to my family and me. It has become familiar to many families in the most destructive ways. It is a persistently cruel and sickening disease that has carved a place in my life that cannot be erased.

My maternal grandmother and great-grandmother both succumbed to breast cancer after a long and tiring fight. My maternal great-grandmother, Ignacia Nápoles, whom I sadly never got the opportunity to meet, was diagnosed with breast cancer at the age of sixty-six and died soon after in communist Cuba, where there was limited healthcare available at the time. My *abuelita* (grandmother in Spanish) was Elena America Bolivar (Nápoles). She was a well-educated, lovely, and enchanting lady. She was born in Cuba in 1933 and was afforded the privileged benefit of studying at Our Lady Star of the Sea in Key West, Florida, for four years as a teenager. She returned to Cuba and attended La Universidad de La Habana, where she pursued a career in pharmacology while she worked full-time for IBM. The misfortune of communism and the perils she faced while having to flee her birth country took a toll on her health. My mom brought Abuelita to live with us at home in Manchester from 2007 until her passing in 2012. She was a strong presence in my life and was very dear to me. I watched the devastatingly agonizing effects of cancer when she was curled up in bed suffering as breast cancer ate away every last second of her life. I remember attending the endless doctor appointments with her and mom just to hear the disappointing diagnoses and hopeless prognoses. It was gut-wrenching to hear the doctor say that my grandmother wasn't going to ever get any better. I could describe in great detail the breast lumps the size of a softball and the obvious pain she endured. I knew we didn't have the money for radiation or treatments. Doctors, my mother, and other healthcare staff did the best they could to keep her alive, while also trying to give her the best quality of life possible.

She passed away four days before her seventy-ninth birthday. I will never forget September 19, 2012. That day, even as a child, changed my life permanently. The cancer had metastasized to her lungs and spread to other major organs, leaving her with almost no cell in her body untouched by the fatal disease.

My mom had a brush with this unrelenting disease as well. She underwent a bilateral mammoplasty in September 2000 to remove questionable tissue from her left breast that was found by a routine mammogram. Later after testing, the tissue was confirmed to be cancerous. There are preventive measures and available routine procedures, but not everyone is fortunate enough to have access to them. Whether because of geographic location or lack of funds, some people cannot receive the necessary medical care. Every life is precious and dignified, and everyone should have access to life-saving procedures.

My paternal great-grandfather, Oather Smith, better known as "papaw" to me, lived a very happy and successful life overall. He was a survivor of colon cancer in his early sixties, before he developed black lung. He worked tirelessly as an electrician in the underground coal mines of Clay County and the surrounding Kentucky counties for thirty-two years to provide the basic necessities and the finer things in life for himself, his wife, and seven children. He was the first person in his community to own a television and to have indoor running water. The coal dust eventually worked its way into his lungs, and he became progressively sicker. He had to involuntarily retire due to the illness and its persistent effects on his health. He was in no shape to work at that point. In fact, he could no longer enjoy his favorite pastime of fishing for walleye at Laurel Lake. He could not enjoy time with his loved ones either. His life was permanently and drastically changed by the destructive disease. I lovingly recall going to see my papaw and the anticipation of the smell of fresh buttermilk biscuits in the morning, which filled the air every time I walked through that screen door. Hearing his voice and climbing up on his lap to watch westerns with him was always my favorite part of my visits. That's what childhood dreams are made of. Cancer wasn't just something he and the family had to live with. It became not only a part of us but of our everyday lives. Cancer is a rough and fearless opponent, to say the least, but it was hard on me too. It scarred my positive outlook on a possible future with my loving papaw. Looking back, I remember moments of seeing everyone putting on a mandatory smile every day. Knowing they were in unbearable physical or emotional pain with no options is what hurts the most.

Is wanting a cure for cancer too much to ask? Of course not! As for the people in my community, it has always been a dream to rise above this disease. At times, it's easily forgotten that cancer is still around and can take a life faster than we can blink. The impact of cancer is frequently ignored. However, it always seemed as though sometimes cancer would whisper in your ear, reminding you that yes, it's still here. It's not giving up without a fight, but neither am I, along with my community.

It has been theorized that chromium is linked to cancer vulnerability and the growth of tumors. So what is chromium? Chromium is a chemical used in different processes. Some of it can be found in dietary supplements, and other particles are used to make stainless steel and other industrial products (such as textiles and even wood products). Chromium-6 can enter drinking water supplies underground, and also through rivers and streams. Frighteningly, chromium-6 is not regulated. Even though the Environmental Protection Agency has set maximum contaminant levels for total chromium in potable drinking water, the level of regulation refers only to nontoxic forms of chromium (not including chromium-6, which is infinitely more toxic).[2] Chromium-6 may be a contaminant of coal mining and thus may be responsible for making many coal miners and residents of coal-mining areas sick.

Cancer impacts Kentuckians in many ways. For some individuals, the geography of Appalachia makes it difficult to travel to receive treatment. Tobacco agriculture and processing are a major source of income for many Kentuckians. Kentucky residents are familiar with the products: cigars, cigarettes, and chewing tobacco ("dip"). The familiarity with these products leaves some with an indelible impression that they are harmless, but they are not. Smoking is the familiar and popular pastime of many people worldwide regardless of age, but it is especially concentrated in the populace of Eastern Kentucky. Many news channels or research studies on common foods and household goods have bombarded viewers with cancer-causing warnings. Recently, a special news broadcast reported that bacon and processed meats can cause cancer. This has intrigued me to do further investigation. While bacon is a rare treat in our household, hotdogs have been an affordable staple in my diet since early adolescence. This sparked immediate concern that I may have been poisoning myself inadvertently. An article on cancer.org stated, "The International Agency for Research on Cancer classifies processed meat as a carcinogen, something that causes cancer. And it classifies red meat as a probable carcinogen, something that probably causes cancer."[3] The article went on to discuss other processed meats that every American enjoys from time to time (such as processed lunch meats and canned meats) during family and event-themed barbecues. It's not hard to find articles on foods and products that "cause cancer"; therefore, it is relatively easy to understand why most people might be dismissive about the subject, declaring, "Oh, everything causes cancer nowadays."

Informing people about the dangers of products that cause cancer has not reduced the incidence of the deadly disease. I have pondered endlessly about possible options to give new insight to the general public about cancer and its prevention. Cancer is preventable in so many cases. It may appear that people are desensitized to cancer, but that is not a reliable reason nor excuse to look the other way. There are currently many fundraisers for cancer research, like Relay for Life, television marathons, and local programs, but that is not enough. Too many people's lives are changed drastically by this disease known as cancer. There are too many types of cancer and too many lives needlessly taken by this attacker. I have taken a vow to dedicate my life and focus my education, just as my mother and so many others have done, to save lives, one at a time. I hope that one day I will be given the opportunity to work as a doctor, helping others who have been seeking the love, dedication, and commitment that I know I can provide. Making cancer screenings and doctor appointments more affordable to those who need them is also something I would love to accomplish in my community. Every life matters, and I would like to have a part in the victorious rejoicing each time cancer is defeated.

My Clay County Home

I am from old dirt roads and swinging bridges
From spring-time garden lillies and honeysuckle vines
I am from banjos and picking guitars in the summer-time festivals
I am from riding ATVs in the mushy mud
I am from fresh flaky biscuits and crispy fried green tomatoes
I am from the old historic log cabins
I am from the smell of fresh baked goods and parade floats on one of
    the county's most important days of the year
I am from cold winter days building glossy white snowmen and drink-
    ing chocolaty marshmallow drinks
I am from loud glistening sparks on a Fourth of July night while cele-
    brating our independence

I am from dark unground tunnels that keep the lights on and stories of those who risk their lives in those tunnels

I am from checkered and different patterned warm cozy quilts on a cold night

I am from cheerful home-welcoming smiling faces

I am from coal miners and cancer survivors

Rachel Collins

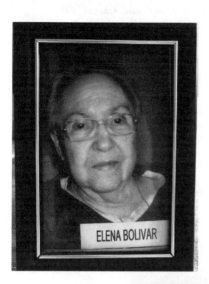
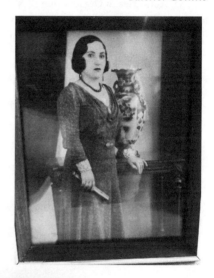

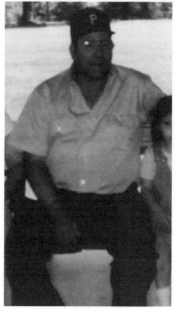

Notes

1. A. Lowrey, "What's the Matter with Eastern Kentucky?" *New York Times,* June 26, 2014, retrieved from https://www.nytimes.com/2014/06/29/magazine/whats-the-matter-with-eastern-kentucky.html.

2. K. Deamer, "Chromium-6 in Tap Water: Why the 'Erin Brockovich' Chemical Is Dangerous," Livescience.com, September 22, 2016, retrieved from https://www.livescience.com/56210-what-is-chromium-6-in-tap-water.html.

3. "World Health Organization Says Processed Meat Causes Cancer," Cancer.org, October 26, 2015, retrieved from https://www.cancer.org/latest-news/world-health-organization-says-processed-meat-causes-cancer.html.

Survivor's Guilt

Andrew Davison

CANCER HAS A complicated history, both in the written records and the hearts and minds of individual persons. Few other diseases have been so familiarized yet stigmatized as cancer. This stigmatization often stems from the assigned blame unique to cancer: lung cancer can frequently be chalked up to a patient's history of smoking, gum cancer can often be traced back to the patient's tobacco use, and many other cancers can develop as a result of exposure to carcinogens. However, in addition to cancers caused by a patient's living habits, there are otherwise healthy people contracting cancer because of genetics, uncontrollable circumstances, and pure random chance.

Regardless of the patient's carcinogenic exposure, there is often a search for blame. Many blame themselves. This can sometimes be an accurate assessment, but the struggle is magnified by self-hate and self-loathing while those patients witness and experience the visceral effects of their bad habits. Many blame others; many blame a religious figure; many blame corporations and factories; many blame a minuscule event or presence in their life—all in the search for something to be held accountable for the patient's misfortune.

The problem that quickly arises is the contradiction between blame assignment and the very nature of cancer. Oftentimes cancer is blameless, developing only as the result of a random mutation of genes, and yet still a multitude of patients seek to condemn themselves with guilt.

When my mother went into remission from her breast cancer, she began to hear the word "survivor." At first, it seems an accurate description for the cancer patients who have gone into remission. These people have often struggled through chemotherapy, through radiation, through medication and surgery, and so much more. Those "survivors" beat cancer because they fought hard against it. The issue that my mother took with the word was that it implied that you could influence the toll that cancer takes on your body. The term, to my mother, meant that those who died struggling with cancer could have survived just like those in remission if only they had just fought harder. It meant that those we have lost to cancer have been lost only because they and their body didn't have what it took to survive cancer.

Of course, we know this isn't true. Many who have succumbed to cancer did everything as prescribed and still died. Other patients have refused the rigorous medical treatment and still went into a miraculous remission. In the question of cancer, willpower matters only until you've done everything your doctors have told you to do. Then some people get luckier than others. It doesn't feel fair, and it doesn't feel right, but it downplays the courage and strength of those lost to the disease.

My mother and I still haven't come up with an alternative to "survivor." While it may imply some falsehoods, it conveys the struggle and hurt experienced during the manifestation and treatment of cancer. Maybe it's not about the word, but its usage. As you call someone in remission a survivor, it will always bring to mind those who aren't. I lost my grandmother to cancer a year after my mother had been diagnosed with breast cancer, and my mother will always think of her mom before she thinks of her own experience.

Similarly, I will always think first of my mother when considering cancer. Although her case was caught early on and her experience was comparatively tame, her treatment still took a toll on her and my family. I remember times when people would visit, and my mother would hurry to cover her bare head. I think now that it was not out of embarrassment but to prevent pity. My mother was still a woman, was still capable of taking care of herself, and the pity that accompanied her diagnosis and treatment diminished that. After all, she was not a survivor.

As for me, I am not a survivor either. I'm just a boy who has seen at least two of his family members lose their lives to cancer and has seen at least three more develop it. My family hails from all regions of the country, but I grew up in Rowan County, Kentucky. My parents both teach at the local university, Morehead State, and I attended the public school in

Rowan County until 2019 when I was accepted into the Gatton Academy at Western Kentucky University. I go to school because I like to learn, but not necessarily because I know how I want to use that learning in the future. My future career and college choices are yet to be made. As a part of the Appalachian Career Training in Oncology (ACTION) Program, I hope to make some choices earlier rather than later, but my experience is more than just about me. It's about helping people.

For a disease as subjective to randomness as cancer, it takes an unusual prevalence in those I know. I have lost both a grandmother and a grandfather to cancer and cancer complications. Beyond that, my mother, two aunts, my other grandmother, and a family friend have all been diagnosed with cancer. Of those five, four of them developed breast cancer. This does not mean, by any measure, that their experiences have been the same. Cancer is very much a personal disease; whereas it may take only a single surgery and a preventative prescription to put some into remission, others endure a lifelong battle that, in some cases, began before I was born. This is partly what makes the disease so terrifying. There is a list of patients with cancer complications that cannot be called short.

While later in life I may not be in a career that directly aims to help people with cancer or promote cancer literacy, I will always remember images of cancer from my childhood. I will remember my grandma's face half-slumped due to a surgery combating her parotid cancer. I will remember walking into a high school bathroom and seeing dipping tobacco splayed in the urinals. I will remember making eye contact with a health teacher as he smoked a cigarette. Maybe I will not be there to witness the effects of some of these acts, but I wish that these consequences would not have to be realized at all.

This is what the ACTION Program allows me to do: as an invested student, I have a streamlined pathway to supplement my cancer education and the influence that I may have on other people. One of the central dogmas of the program is the focus on Kentucky—or the more encompassing Appalachian region. Kentucky is a leading state in cancer development and cancer-related deaths.[1] I have grown up and have seen family and friends suffer from cancer in Kentucky. I have been reared in the public school system where I have seen budding Kentucky citizens willfully expose themselves to carcinogens. Finding a way to prevent Kentucky youths from exposing themselves to carcinogens is nearly an impossible task.

One of the main reasons Kentucky is so disproportionately hit with cancer (in particular, lung cancer) is the long history of the importance of tobacco in the state economy. Even after removing government-backed tobacco price supports, instituting a system of tobacco crop quotas, limiting tobacco sales to people over age eighteen, and mandating tobacco bans in public places in many communities, Kentucky *still* has the second highest rate of tobacco production in the United States, after North Carolina.[2] Tobacco products are known and well-documented carcinogens, and despite efforts to combat tobacco use in the state, modern products, such as e-cigarettes and vapes, facilitate the continued and unfortunate trend among youth who would otherwise not participate in the more traditional vehicles for nicotine and its associated carcinogens.

An important movement in Kentucky, reflected by the ACTION Program, is the shift away from an agrarian economy. One particular industry that is expanding and will provide jobs for many is the healthcare industry, as regional hospitals are built in more rural areas of the state that did not previously have readily available access to professional healthcare.

The ACTION Program is representative of this economic shift in many ways. Clearly, it exemplifies the expansion of the Kentucky healthcare industry. It also works to encourage a new generation of Kentucky citizens to dedicate their lives to a career focused on the good health of Kentuckians. Although I do come from a county with a regional hospital, many of my peers do not, and ACTION works excellently to show the importance of available healthcare.

However, regional hospitals do have their limitations. Everyone I know who has been diagnosed with cancer while living in Kentucky was treated at the Markey Cancer Center. As I took a tour through University of Kentucky buildings during my ACTION Orientation Day, my mother, who had had her breast cancer treated there years earlier, could still tell me the names of buildings and point out the rooms where she received chemotherapy. The UK Healthcare complex has an important leading role in Kentucky, and I am proud to be able to take part in expanding its positive influence throughout the state.

The experience that the ACTION Program provides and will continue to provide for me will be invaluable in my future. I know that because it cultivates so many separate areas of my personality and academics, it will have an impact on my future choices and career decisions. In the program,

I have bonded with roommates, practiced researching procedures, and learned a computer programming language, and I have tried to use every moment to better myself and what I can hope to achieve. The ACTION Program has broadened my horizons and given me so many opportunities that were not previously even in my periphery.

Although it may not seem like it, I am appreciative for the way I was raised in my home county. My parents allowed me to meet educated people that, at first, gave me a better perspective on cancer as some of them fought through it. That view was qualified later by a more personal experience with my grandma, as I had never known someone who had died as a result of cancer. Up until that moment, cancer had felt like a toll on the turnpike of life, but I never thought that it could be so expensive. These contrasting ideals—one downplaying the seriousness and one bordering on the hyperbolic—together created the approach I needed to be sensitive and rational about cancer. ACTION has only refined that, giving me the utmost respect for those working against the course of the disease and its development. In my life, I hope to accomplish something as noteworthy and as positive for the people around me as those researchers and doctors have.

Above all, I hope that I can become a positive influence on the world around me. Oncology may be how I do that, or maybe the social skills developed during ACTION will allow me to create joy on a more personal level for others. Whatever it may be, I will remember growing up in Kentucky. I will never forget my grandma, who always influenced those around her for the better. I will value every moment with my aunt, who has been battling metastasized breast cancer since I was a child. The harrowing tobacco culture of school will surely never escape me, and I know that I will always regret standing by while my peers became addicted to those harmful substances. I hope that the measure of my life will be taken in what I have done for others, and I hope that I measure up well.

Notes

1. CDC, "USCS Data Visualizations," November 2018, accessed June 25, 2019, from https://gis.cdc.gov/Cancer/USCS/DataViz.html.

2. WorldAtlas.com, "Tobacco Production by State," 2017, accessed June 25, 2019, from https://www.worldatlas.com/articles/states-leading-the-way-in-us-tobacco-production.html.

Careless Cancer

Holly Dickens

WHEN I WAS introduced to the Appalachian Career Training in Oncology (ACTION) Program at my school by the program coordinator, Chris Prichard, I could not stop thinking about how perfect the program would be for me. I started my application essay as soon as I got home from school. There was not a day that went by that I did not think about how great it would be if I got accepted, and to my delight, I was accepted.

My name is Holly Dickens. I am from Rowan County, Kentucky, and I attend Rowan County Senior High School. I have wanted to go into the medical field for as long as I can remember, and I have always loved science. In 2014, my experience with transverse myelitis showed me the effects healthcare providers can have on patients and their families. My doctor was a symbol of hope to me because he was the only person who understood what was wrong with me. Being able to help and give hope to people in possibly the worst situations of their lives is something that I would love to be able to do. Also, through AP biology in my sophomore year, after doing experiments in class, I learned that I am interested in research and that a combined career in research and healthcare was an option. It would be so rewarding to help people directly through treatment, as well as being able to help from the root of the problem through research.

My first experience with cancer was with my mom's good friend. Growing up, I was pretty close with my mom's friends since I was frequently around them at her work. I do not remember much because I was young, but I remember the impact it had on my mom and her friends. It is hard to comprehend the thought of losing such a close friend. She was diagnosed with breast cancer, which had then metastasized to other parts of her body.

My mom and I went to visit her when she did not have much time left. It was a moment that I have always remembered, and I probably will always remember it. It was the first time that I had personally witnessed the impact of a cancer-caused death. Moreover, there is a picture of my mom's friend with cancer at the beach, which was somewhere she wanted to go before she passed, that is still stuck in my mind. This experience introduced to me how truly devastating cancer can be to everyone involved.

A few years ago, the person who has always mowed our lawn was diagnosed with cancer. He has had his lawn-mowing business for a long time, and when he found out he had cancer, it made him think about changing his career to something that would be more compliant with the possible needs of his diagnosis. Cancer uproots people's lives, makes them think about their new future, and definitely does not take into account what people love and are passionate about. It causes an unwanted, abrupt change in people's lives due to a mere accident, a mutation.

When I was around eleven, my aunt was diagnosed with leukemia, which runs in her family. Fortunately, it is not a bad type of leukemia, but it is still scary to know that other people in her family could later be diagnosed as well. When cancer is in a family's genetics, it is bittersweet to watch the family grow. In addition, when cancer is in a family's genetics, children who do not know their family's health history are not aware that cancer could be in their future. When my parents were at a car dealership one day, the salesman told us that he had had colon cancer a couple years ago. Prior to knowing he had cancer, he was someone who did not know his father, and he successfully set out to meet him. He found that his father had colon cancer, and it ran in the family. So after putting off the dreaded colonoscopy, he finally decided to have one, and his doctor found that he had colon cancer. Thankfully, they caught it early enough that he became cancer free after chemotherapy treatment. His story made me think about how silent cancer can be until it is too late, and how it is such a miracle to be able to save someone's life.

Just recently, my friend's grandmother was diagnosed with a tumor on her pituitary gland. She had been having severe headaches for months, and that discrete symptom was passed over as a sinus issue until her doctor ordered a CT scan, which revealed the true cause. Such an unexpected diagnosis caused a lot of stress for my friend and her family, and the necessary surgeries placed even more stress and worry on them. Cancer enters people's lives abruptly when the seemingly normal symptoms of common conditions turn out to be this jarring disease.

A couple years ago in my community, there was a big fundraiser for a former student of Rowan County High School who was diagnosed with cancer. Everyone knew about the cause, and everyone was trying to help. My school in particular helped a lot with popularizing the cause. At basketball games and football games, we would wear the shirts that the family was selling for the fundraiser. It was amazing to see the whole community being involved in such a great cause and how hard everyone worked to help the family. It would be great to see communities everywhere be this strong in assisting those with cancer.

When living in the many rural areas of Kentucky, residents have little exposure to information about cancer. There are not many programs that inform communities about the important causes of cancer and ways to prevent cancer. Without information about the causes of cancer and without emphasis on the importance of cancer screenings, Kentuckians are more susceptible to cancer because they are blind to it. As many people are aware, it is a stereotype for Kentuckians to excessively use tobacco products. Although this is a stereotype and obviously does not apply to all Kentucky citizens, this stereotype did not come about without reason. Many Kentuckians use significantly more tobacco products compared to the national average, among both adults and minors.[1] Due to the lack of information given to people about the dangers of tobacco use, they continue to use until it is too late. Tobacco is a major cause of cancer that can easily be prevented, but people choose to still use it. People need to understand that their actions can cause them to get cancer. Information about the impact of tobacco use on people's health is crucial.

Furthermore, people need to be reminded of the importance of cancer screenings. It is crucial for cancer to be caught early to better the prognosis. For many people, it is scary to get screened for cancer. What if you unexpectedly get diagnosed and have a short time to live? What would happen to your family? What would be the cost of treatment? Many people experience this anxiety, and in turn, they do not get checked for cancer. For instance, colonoscopies are a type of cancer screening that many people put off. No one wants to take off work to prepare for a screening that seems unnecessary. If you do not have symptoms, how could you have cancer? There is a big push for people of ages fifty to seventy-five to get a colonoscopy, but the effort is only partially successful. Again, if more information about cancer and the importance of cancer screenings was provided to people, it would be helpful in preventing and catching cancer early. With the help of the outreach activities we will plan as part of the ACTION Program, we will provide important information about cancer, the treatments for cancer, and the prevention of cancer to our communities.

Along with the need for informing people about cancer is the need for physicians to be able to find the early symptoms of cancer that are often overlooked. There are many stories about people who had early symptoms of cancer whose symptoms were overlooked at their normal checkups, like my friend's grandmother and the car salesman, for example. People often blame their doctors for missing these symptoms, but the real blame is on the lack of attention given to the early symptoms, which are often very mild. For instance, in colon cancer, an early symptom that could easily be overlooked is abdominal pain, which could be associated with many other diagnoses. We need to find a better way to detect these symptoms so that they are not brushed off and so the cancer does not get a chance to worsen.

Everywhere, not just in Kentucky, cancer is a *bad* word. It is associated with death, sickness, and sadness. That is all we see of cancer. If we were exposed to all of the positive news about cancer—effective treatments, cancer screenings that caught cancer early and saved a person's life, and advancements in treatment—there could be a better outlook on life with cancer. People would have less anxiety toward cancer screenings, which could help create more success stories. As more time passes, cancer can become a less intimidating disease in the light of the new treatments and preventions, and people deserve to know about these advancements and victories.

Notes

1. CDC, "Behavioral Risk Factor Surveillance System (2016), 2018 Kentucky tobacco use fact sheet," retrieved from truthinitiative.org. Also CDC, "Youth Risk Behavior System (2017), 2018 Kentucky tobacco use fact sheet," retrieved from truthinitiative.org.

Cancer
A War on the Home Front

Zachary Hall

WHAT TRULY DEFINES a person's life? Is it the air they breathe, the clothes on their backs, or the place they live? In all of my understanding, I've come to realize that it is not truly a person's success that defines their life, but the hardships, defeats, and roads they've walked that truly define how they live. These hard times shape not only that one person, but all those around them.

There are many evils that prevail in our world, but there is one that has claimed many lives—too many. This evil is cancer, and it is a horrific monster that feeds upon the weak and the strong, attacking and killing without remorse. Here in Southeastern Kentucky (in fact, all of Kentucky), that monster has had its fill, and it continues its gluttonous feeding every day. This epidemic is so large in this area that not only does everyone know someone who has or has had cancer, but a large majority of people have had cancer affect their own family. I have had numerous family members affected by cancer: both of my great-grandfathers, both of my great-grandmothers, my cousin, and my grandfather. Many people look upon this and think of sorrow and sickness, but I look at their experiences and see strength and perseverance.

My name is Zachary Hall, a native of Letcher County, and my bloodline is filled with "Cancer Warriors" who have both won and lost against this monstrosity. I am ready to take up arms against this evil and fight it on the front lines, so to speak, in this "war" that has gone on for too long.

My desire to go into the medical field and to focus on oncology is fueled by the experiences my family has gone through with cancer. It has turned my desire into a sense of duty, an act of vengeance against this plague.

Through this, I hope to eradicate this evil so that families will never have to suffer the losses I have. As I previously alluded to, many members of my family have had cancer. My grandmother's father, William Clayton Witt, had very aggressive testicular cancer. He defeated this cancer, but five years later, the cancer recurred, but this time it had metastasized to his brain and was incurable. He later died as a result but served as an inspiration to us all through his valiant fighting and perseverance, qualities that can inspire all who struggle, with cancer or other challenges. His wife, my great-grandmother Dorothy Witt, died of lung cancer, which was also a challenging ordeal given that she had had one lung transplant and lived with that for a while. Her bravery, even through the pain, is yet another example to follow and is an inspiration to me.

On my grandfather's side, my great-grandfather James M. Caudill Jr. had colon cancer, which was in the exact same spot where his mother, Atha B. Caudill, had had cancer. The surgeon said that he had "never seen anything like it," referring to their cancers' being exactly identical. Was their cancer merely a coincidence or something more? The possibilities interest and terrify me. Both survived, however. My great-grandmother Betty Wynkoop Caudill had very aggressive breast cancer. The cancer metastasized to the liver, and eventually to the brain, which would lead to her death. Betty's cancer was the one that has had the greatest effect on me because I can remember that one in detail. At the time, all I knew was that cancer was a bad sickness. I thought that it was like a cold and that all people would get over it. After her death, cancer had a brand-new meaning to me. The rides in her red Mustang with the top down were now nothing more than a memory. Her smile that could light up a room was now pale and lifeless. Cancer had delivered her right into the hands of Death as if they had greeted each other as old friends. I learned then that cancer was not just a sickness. It was a plague; it was sorrow, and it was pain.

From that moment on, cancer crept into my life more and more and eventually became something I saw around every corner, both here at home and everywhere else. It took hold of my grandfather Barry Caudill as he developed skin cancer, but he caught it in time and had the mass removed. Cancer also found a home in my cousin Juanita Spangler as she developed breast cancer and fought for her life, eventually defeating this evil.

Cancer has affected me very closely—too closely. You could say I have a personal vendetta against cancer, a score to settle with it for all the pain it has caused my family and everyone else it has touched. This outrageous number of family members affected by cancer is very high, which may lead people to believe that something is afoot here in Southeastern Kentucky, which brings us to my next focus: why I believe cancer impacts Kentuckians so harshly.

If you ever travel to Letcher County and ask about the cancer problem here and what people think causes it, I guarantee that almost everyone you ask will tell you that it is "in the water." I have heard many people, old and young, say this exact statement. So when a multitude of people say the exact same thing, why would you not give them any credence? If you have to describe the basis of Letcher County's economy, it would have been coal, the keywords being "would have been." The economy in Letcher County can now be described in a new way: "filled with poverty," which I will discuss further.

Letcher County's economy was seemingly completely reliant upon the coal-mining industry given the surplus of coal that was found in the mountains of Letcher County and the surrounding counties around the state, which led to the mining of coal seemingly everywhere in these parts. There are several ways that coal mining has been linked to cancer over the years. One way is the inhalation of dust during coal mining, which can lead to lung cancer and can also lead to a condition known as "Black Lung." Given that coal mining was, and still is in some places, the predominant industry in Eastern Kentucky, many people are coal miners. Hypothetically, if each of these coal miners worked for many years in these mines, breathing in that deadly dust, wouldn't there be an influx of cancer patients and fatalities due to cancer? Sounds scary, right? Now, what if I told you that the truly scary part is that none of this was hypothetical at all? That is the scary part. The rates of cancer in these regions tell the truth of how deadly coal mining has been on the residents of Kentucky, especially Eastern Kentucky. As to how coal mining affects the water, many residents of Letcher County and the neighboring counties have said cancer is caused by all of the inlets and streams coming out of mines, carrying chemicals, sulfur, and many other things. Companies and other people who are financially and emotionally driven choose to avoid this topic because they are trying to revive the coal industry or because they think that there is nothing wrong with the water. In my opinion, however, I believe that our water may very well be contaminated by the coal mines. If so, then the everyday water we cook with, drink, and bathe in may be slowly killing us all, which is both terrifying and extremely unsafe.

Now to refer back to the economy. As the coal economy collapses, so does the economy of Letcher County and many other counties. The state of the economy when it comes to cancer can literally mean life or death. I believe that another reason that these Kentucky regions have the highest cancer rates and highest cancer mortality rates of anywhere else in America is due to the shattered economies that all of these communities have.[1] A poor economy leads to poor citizens, which means that a lot of people don't have enough money for proper healthcare. Due to this lack of money, many people can't pay for their treatments if they have cancer or refuse treatments in order to provide for their family instead. I have known several people that could not buy medication because they wouldn't be able to buy food for their family if they did. So now we see how the two epidemics of Eastern Kentucky, cancer and poverty, go hand in hand in destroying people and families all across Kentucky. However, even though the prospects look dim when looking at these two evils, there is hope on how we can address cancer in our state.

According to the National Cancer Institute, Kentucky is the nation's leader in cancer rates and deaths due to cancer. In addition to this startling statistic, the Appalachian region of Kentucky from which I hail is affected worse than any other region in Kentucky and is in need of drastic help. There are many solutions that I believe could help address the rates of cancer in Kentucky. One that I strongly believe in is making people more aware of cancer and what options they have. In Eastern Kentucky and other rural parts, many people are not educated about cancer or what treatment options they have. For example, if a person has random spots show up on their skin, they may not think anything of it, but it may very well be skin cancer, which could be deadly if left untreated. These spots can appear in a variety of forms such as a simple mole, freckle, or any kind of skin blotch. However, if that same person were educated on what different types of cancer there are, what they look like, and what treatment options there are, theoretically, that person would be more likely to consult a doctor, and the cancer may be caught early and removed. Education is vital to our society and can reroute our brain to take more precautionary measures, leading to a decrease in fatalities due to cancer. People can be educated via social media, awareness assemblies, paper and television ads, and even volunteer classes that teach the facts about cancer.

Another very important solution lies within the Markey Cancer Center's Appalachian Career Training in Oncology (ACTION) Program itself. This program, which I am proudly a part of, is teaching and training future oncology professionals to not just treat cancer, but to defeat it completely and maybe even find a cure. The future is no longer filled with impossibilities, only possibilities—limitless ones. Through the knowledge acquired, cancer doesn't stand a chance. We have been searching for a cure for cancer for many years, and our best shot at defeating it is through programs like the ACTION Program that teaches people how to defeat cancer, to be creative, and to not give up so that the blood, sweat, and tears in pursuit of a cure will amount to one. We need to focus on fresh minds, creativity, and dedication from our world's youth to step up and give fresh new ideas in defeating this monster. The ACTION Program gives a close-up account of what cancer is and how it can be fought. This training and the interest that it sparks is invaluable, and we participants are eager to take up the mantle of our mentors already, not for fame, not for fortune, but for the well-being of humankind.

My family's struggle with cancer, my community's struggle with cancer, and the opportunity I have with the ACTION Program have further fueled my desire to work in the medical field, particularly as a surgical oncologist. My life has been filled with many people who have always inspired me to do my best, but my main drive is humanity. I have no greater joy than helping others. The opportunity to save lives and being able to have the education to do so is like a dream come true. To answer my previous question on what defines a person's life, it is their hardships, but it is also how that person and their experiences affect and shape that person. Eleanor Roosevelt once said, "You gain strength, courage, and confidence by every experience in which you really stop to look fear in the face. You are able to say to yourself, 'I lived through this horror. I can take the next thing that comes along.'" Mrs. Roosevelt's quote really makes you think. Think of what cancer survivors go through, all of the pain, suffering, anxiety, and panic, and they lived through it all. Can you imagine that strength? They are my role models. They continuously shape me into a better person. They have stared right into Death's face and told him, "Not today." They have told cancer to pack its bags, that it has no home in their body anymore. If a person can go through that much and still be smiling at the end of the day, then that shows you that they are a warrior. That is the type of spirit we must have when dealing with cancer and searching for a cure. Whether we are in a lab, removing tumors in surgery, or even teaching a class about cancer, we must keep that same warrior spirit. That is the strength, courage, and confidence that can defeat any evil, so why should cancer be any different? I am the future. You are the future. We all are the future. It doesn't matter where you're from or who you are, we all have the potential to do anything we set our minds to, even defeating cancer. If we keep that same warrior spirit that the Cancer Warriors all around the world and even here in Kentucky have, then cancer doesn't stand a chance.

Notes

1. National Cancer Institute, "State Cancer Profiles," https://statecancerprofiles.cancer.gov.

A Monster That Kills

Abigail Isaacs

MALCOLM X ONCE said, "Education is the passport to the future, for tomorrow belongs to those who prepare for it today." My name is Abigail Isaacs, and I am currently enrolled in the Appalachian Career Training in Oncology (ACTION) Program through the University of Kentucky Markey Cancer Center. I was born on September 28, 2003, and was raised in a small town where I'm still living today. I am an upcoming junior at Garrard County High School in Garrard County, Kentucky. I play soccer for the varsity team as a Lady Lion. This past soccer season I was injured throughout multiple games; I eventually found out that I had fractured my kneecap. After weeks of waiting to see an orthopedic doctor, my fracture had healed, but I still couldn't walk. From multiple MRIs and physical tests, I soon learned that my MPFL (medial patella femur ligament) was torn, as well as my meniscus, and I had broken off part of my cartilage in my knee. After nine months of physical therapy, I should be able to return not only to my soccer family, but to my forever sport. Other than sports, I'm highly involved with academics as well. In the summer of 2019, I attended the Rogers Scholars Program. This is a program through the Center of Rural Development that provides leadership and college scholarship opportunities to help upcoming high school juniors better prepare for their future. My future career has always been to work in the pediatric field and to specialize in oncology. Having a greater understanding of cancer today makes me yearn to work in the field where our population is greatly affected.

Cancer runs in my family on both my mom's and my dad's side. There are about six different cancers that my family has seen in different ancestors: brain, skin, prostate, lung, colon, and breast cancers. This disease has always been a burden on my family, and still is. When I was young, I thought the word *cancer* was just some type of sickness that everyone gets, just like a cold. As a child, I soon found that the true meaning of cancer is that it is an epidemic. My granny told me to think of cancer as a bulldozer, tearing down a house that was once standing. I came to the realization that this was no cold that someone catches; it's a monster that comes into your life, just like the monsters you see on television. I never knew that learning the meaning of this word would change everything.

"Cancer is a word, not a sentence," said John Diamond. When I was five, I lost one of the most important people in my life. My nanny was my best friend, and not a day goes by that I don't wish I could see her one more time. She was diagnosed with small-cell carcinoma located in her lungs in May 2008, which then metastasized to multiple places in her body. Small-cell carcinoma is an aggressive form of lung cancer, which commonly occurs in smokers. My brother never got to meet my nanny, but I will always tell him how great of a woman she was. The day that cancer finally took her life was in June 2008. I remember every detail of that day. The day she died, my mom came to school to pick me up, and all I remember was being confused about why I had to leave so early. She then told me on the way to my nanny's house that she was no longer with us. She had gone to see my papaw Butch in Heaven, who died from cancer as well. I was so angry at the world for taking away my precious nanny. In reality, it was the monster we call cancer that had taken her life way too soon. Along with my nanny, her husband, my papaw Butch, was diagnosed with small-cell carcinoma. His cancer continued to metastasize into his kidneys and his brain. He was given two months to live, and he passed exactly on the two-month mark of his diagnosis. I never got to meet my papaw Butch because the disease had taken a man that everyone knew as a wonderful person before I was born. Along with them was my papaw Sheperson, who always called me "that girl." He was a Kentucky State policeman and firefighter who would give you the shirt off his back. In 2007, he was diagnosed with prostate cancer, which metastasized and forced him to have seventeen inches of his large intestine removed, and he had to have a colostomy bag afterward. This procedure slowed down the rate of cancer that was growing within his body, but then the doctors soon found out that his cancer had continued to spread. His lymph nodes and his brain were rapidly taken over by cancer. The day he was admitted into the hospital, he couldn't find his way home, and my grandma soon knew that something was terribly wrong. On July 5, 2010, doctors had taken him back to perform a PET scan. They quit counting the polyps at seventeen because there was no way anyone could survive with an increasing number of polyps. These are abnormal tissue growths that most often look like small, flat bumps or tiny crests within the skin. He later died in the hospital, and he never had a chance to make it home. Alongside my papaw Sheperson, my nanny, and my papaw Butch, my great-aunt developed breast cancer, which resulted in her having a double mastectomy. In the blink of an eye, the doctors found that the cancer had spread into her brain. She never stopped fighting the battle that cancer had brought upon her. She defeated one of the hardest battles she ever had to fight and ultimately overcame cancer. This urges me even more to search for a cure for this deadly disease. Even though cancer has taken away some of the most influential people in my life, it has also brought us closer in the times we had with them.

According to the American Cancer Society, "Kentucky has the highest overall mortality and incidence rate for cancer in the United States." In Kentucky there were an estimated 26,000 new cases of cancer in 2019, the most commonly occurring types being lung, breast, and colon cancers.[1] Tobacco products and e-cigarettes are among the most purchased items in gas stations and convenience stores. Not only are adults purchasing these items, but teens are as well. With an increasing amount of nicotine inhaled in people's lungs, there is a higher chance for them to develop cancer in different stages of their life. Each cigarette taken into your body damages DNA in the cells in your body, and when the same cells are damaged numerous times, they can develop cancer.

In addition to tobacco products affecting the lives of people in Kentucky, there is little to no education on screening for cancer. Screenings can help doctors detect and treat different types of cancer early before there are any symptoms. Early detections will show the types of tissues being affected by cancer, and finding a cancer early can improve one's chances of survival. Kentucky´s cancer rate is progressively becoming worse every day. Visiting your doctor regularly can help detect cancer early, and for most cancers, earlier detection can make treatment easier on you and your body. People are not aware of the mortality cancer brings upon us a whole. We all need to come together and find a cure for this monster that has been taking away lives for many years.

The American Cancer Society states that Kentucky has many cancer risk factors.[2] Kentuckians need to come together to slow the rate of cancer growth among us. By enforcing rules and regulations for tobacco products, we can decrease the demand for these substances. Nicotine is an addiction that continues to be fed, especially when teens are pressured to try tobacco products. In the end, this addiction takes over your body and causes multiple dilemmas. Other than cigarettes, Juuls, e-cigs, and vapes are increasingly found among teens in schools. They are easy to hide, and most teachers don't assume that kids would carry items such as these in their pockets. Although not using such products can be a lifestyle choice one can make to prevent cancer, there are still many people who smoke and use tobacco. Every inhale of vapor filled with nicotine is damaging the cells in your lungs. According to the Centers for Disease Control and Prevention, 480,000 people in the United States die each year because of smoking, which means this habit causes one out of every five deaths, yet schools do not have any routine checks or classes showing the major outcomes of such "trends."[3] Your diet and the way you consume certain foods can play a large role in your cancer risk as well; obesity is linked to many cancers. Skin cancer is one of the most common types of cancer and is one that can be prevented. Regardless of the season or weather, you should always wear a broad-spectrum sunscreen. Exercising can maintain the body in multiple ways and ultimately prevent certain diseases, such as cancer. By the time symptoms appear, cancer may have begun to spread and be harder to treat. There are multiple ways to prevent cancer, and more research is needed to better understand all the causes of cancer. Overall, we need to better inform our communities about how one major screen could potentially save a life, and we need education efforts to show others that cancer is truly a monster.

As a person who has been affected so deeply by cancer, I know there are multiple things that I can do to prevent cancer. Residents of Kentucky, I strongly believe, should put broadcasts out into the news showing the risks that you may face daily. Without having a better understanding of cancer, you could soon put yourself at a higher risk for cancer cells to invade your body. Overall, I know how deeply this can affect people, for I have seen the major destruction cancer plays in our lives. You could say that cancer is just a disease, but it has become more than that; it is now a behemoth, a monster that kills.

Notes

1. American Cancer Society, "Cancer Facts & Statistics," https://cancerstatisticscenter. cancer.org/#!/state/Kentucky.

2. Ibid.

3. Centers for Disease Control and Prevention, *Tobacco-Related Mortality,* January 17, 2018, retrieved from Centers for Disease Control and Prevention, https://www.cdc.gov/ tobacco/data_statistics/fact_sheets/fast_facts/index.htm. Also Centers for Disease Control and Prevention, :Tobacco related mortality," https://www.cdc.gov/tobacco/data_statistics/ fact_sheets/health_effects/tobacco_related_mortality/index.htm.

The Worst of Both Worlds

Shahid Jabbar

CANCER IS A disease that anyone can get. It has many varieties, and it ruins families. It causes people to suffer and relationships to fall apart. I am lucky that no one in my family has ever had to suffer from cancer. But what worries me is that the people of Pakistan, my home country, are very prone to cancer and different diseases.

Hi, my name is Shahid Jabbar. Currently, I am a sophomore at Bath County High School. I belong to an Asian family, and I am from Pakistan. I am the first person in my family who is going to graduate high school and attend college. I moved to the United States when I was six years old, and since then, my family has been moving back and forth. My family and I live in a rural community within the Appalachian Mountains. Bath County has a population of 12,378 people, spread out in three main cities: Owingsville, Sharpsburg, and Salt Lick. I have kept perfect attendance and a perfect 4.0 GPA for two years now. I also participate in many different clubs at school like HOSA (Health Occupation Students of America), FBLA (Future Business Leaders of America), writing club, and golf club. All of these clubs have taught me the skills of the real world. For example, HOSA has taught me the skills that could save a life, like CPR and the Heimlich maneuver, while FBLA has taught me money-management skills. My hobbies out of school are playing table tennis and video games, reading fiction and suspenseful books, and cooking. I am fluent in two languages, English and Urdu.

When I was a freshman in high school, I was selected into the Upward Bound program at Morehead State University. This program taught me a lot of life skills and about college life. The summer of my freshman year, I had a chance to travel to Morehead State University and live on campus to learn about college.

When I graduate from college, my dream is to become a cardiologist. I know that becoming a cardiologist will be hard, but that doesn't mean it is impossible. I plan to graduate early from high school, attend Morehead State University for my bachelor's degree in chemistry, and then attend the University of Kentucky to earn my medical degree. After that, I plan to attend residency at the University of Kentucky to get certified for cardio-thoracic surgery. I believe that I can achieve my goal because I am a very confident, hard-working person, and I have high self-esteem. Although my education will be expensive, I plan to pay for college by earning scholar-ships and applying for federal grants.

Once I become a cardiovascular surgeon, I plan to travel back to my home country. Pakistan is a "third-world" country, and I plan to start a free healthcare system for the poor and provide them with the best facili-ties possible. Afterward, I plan to come back to the United States to open clinics in rural areas to provide healthcare to the people who don't have access to it or cannot afford it. I plan to do this by getting medical grants and investors to fund different clinics in Pakistan. I also plan to generate some income here in the United States, which will be used to benefit the people of Pakistan.

My parents have played an essential role in my life and my education. Every day, even now, my family encourages me to learn something new and to improve the skills that I already have. My parents have always want-ed me to be successful and have a fantastic career as a doctor. It was my grandfather's wish for me to become a doctor, and I am going to fulfill his dreams and try my best to succeed.

My family and I settled in the United States in 2014. Pakistan is my home country, and right now, the people of Pakistan are suffering due to the absence of healthcare. The government is corrupt, and the leaders are taking care of themselves instead of the country. Most people in Pakistan are uneducated because people can't afford preschool, kindergarten, mid-dle school, high school, and college fees. Most of the population are either farmers or business owners. Some of the leading causes of death in Pakistan are heart disease, stroke, lower respiratory disorders, pre-term birth com-plications, and various types of cancers.[1] All of these diseases are caused by the absence of healthcare and poor hygiene. If there are hospitals, they are made for profit. Poor people can't afford healthcare, and they have no choice but to suffer. The government doesn't provide clean water, food, or shelter for people who can't afford it. Every day, the electricity goes out for about four to six hours. On a typical summer day, the average temperature is about 34 degrees Celsius, which is around 94 degrees Fahrenheit. Some people have to travel long distances to get fresh and clean water. Most of the time, people die from thirst and hunger because they can't afford food. The government plays an essential role in this. The officials can raise the prices of gasoline or bread at any time because they are profiting from it.

I feel that a major cause of death in Pakistan is lower respiratory disorders and kidney failures, which are caused by unsanitary water. Most people in Pakistan are farmers, and most of the farmers are either right at the poverty level or below it. Poverty is causing people to develop lung and lower respiratory cancer because many citizens spend what little money they have on cigarettes to relieve stress or fight depression. In the long term, this causes asthma, lung cancer, and many more diseases. The government of Pakistan should educate people more about medicine. They should create free local health clinics and try to increase the annual income for the people.

The Pakistani government is corrupt and misleading, and the people suffer for it. This needs to be fixed by the people. There should be more resources available to people like free education, more local hospitals, Medicare, clean water, and food. Overall, the people of Pakistan should be in control of the government, not the officials, and the United Nations should also get involved to provide help to the people who need it.

According to the World Cancer Research Fund, the United States is listed as one of the top five countries with the highest rates of cancer.[2] Within the United States, Kentucky is the top-ranking state with the most significant number of lung cancer cases recorded every year, which causes about 185 out of every 100,000 deaths.[3]

The most common cancer type in Kentucky is lung and bronchus cancer.[4] This is because the people of Kentucky are uneducated about cancer, especially in Eastern Kentucky. People live in rural areas of the Appalachian Mountains and are unaware of the diseases and the necessary medical knowledge related to cancer.

Poverty also plays a big part in Kentucky. Most of the population works at the minimum wage, which is $7.25 an hour. The minimum wage causes people not to be able to have any medical insurance. Limited access to medical assistance also causes people not to be screened for cancer or any diseases. Because of the poverty in Kentucky, the lifestyle of people has changed. People smoke, chew tobacco, and drink alcohol, which in the long term can all lead to lung and bronchus cancer. The life expectancy of Kentuckians is five years shorter than that of the rest of the United States.[5] In the year 2017, the top three causes of death in Kentucky were heart disease, cancer, and chronic lower respiratory disease.[6] This includes heart attacks, heart failure, lung cancer, breast cancer, COPD, asthma, and other related diseases.

For people to become aware of cancer and different types of diseases, they need to be educated. This can be done in several different ways. The ACTION (Appalachian Career Training in Oncology) Program is one way to teach the future generation and provide them with knowledge about cancer and the causes of it. For example, students in the ACTION Program are given the opportunity to shadow doctors and labs related to cancer and its cure. Hospitals like the University of Kentucky and Baptist Health should host workshops around the Appalachian area to train people and educate them about medical terminology, rules and regulations, improvements in medicine, treatment of cancer, and medical education in general. This will also teach them about the signs and symptoms of diseases and their treatments.

Additionally, the Kentucky government should open more rural clinics, providing cheap or free care for all people. There should be fundraising for cancer patients, and professionals should be available for people to talk to about cancer. Colleges and healthcare facilities should have public educational events and seminars free of charge to educate the community. Places like health districts and clinics should pass out posters to raise awareness. There should be more free substance-abuse and cancer-diagnosing clinics available to the people. The minimum wage should be raised so that the people can make an excellent average yearly income and be able to afford medical care for themselves and their families. The taxes on substances like cigarettes and alcohol should be higher than usual to decrease the demand. There should be fines if people are smoking or drinking in a public place and harming others. All of these things would cause people to become more educated and be more cautious about smoking and drinking. This will also encourage people to get screened for common cancers like lung, bladder, kidney, breast, and lower respiratory cancers. In the end, educating people will help them stop smoking and get screened for cancers, thus preventing cancer or detecting it at an early stage. Furthermore, the measures discussed above can be implemented to allow cancer treatments to become more accessible than before. By taking the steps explained above, we the people can slow down or even stop cancer from growing by finding a cure.

Overall, the healthcare conditions in Pakistan and Kentucky are very similar. The people are uneducated about medicine, and there is a meager number of hospitals available for the people to access. The wages for the people in both places are very low. This causes people to stress more and gain bad habits like smoking. This should be fixed by increasing the minimum wage and providing better healthcare to more people.

Notes

1. A. Mwaniki, *Leading Causes of Death in Pakistan,* July 30, 2019, retrieved from World Atlas, https://www.worldatlas.com/articles/leading-causes-of-death-in-pakistan. html. Also Global Cancer Observatory, *Global Cancer Data by Country,* 2018, retrieved from World Cancer Research Fund, https://www.wcrf.org/dietandcancer/cancer-trends/ data-cancer-frequency-country.

2. American Cancer Society, *Cancer Statistics Center,* 2018, retrieved from American Cancer Society, https://cancerstatisticscenter.cancer.org/?_ga=2.230685724.1272622378 .1564585052–2078621239.1563578442#!/state/Kentucky.

3. Wikipedia, *List of U.S. states and territories by life expectancy,* November 2019, retrieved from Wikipedia, https://en.m.wikipedia.org/wiki/List_of_U.S._states_and_territories_by_life_expectancy.

4. Ibid.

5. Centers for Disease Control and Prevention, *National Center for Health Statistics,* April 11, 2018, retrieved from Centers for Disease Control and Prevention, https://www. cdc.gov/nchs/pressroom/states/kentucky/kentucky.htm.

6. Ibid.

Kentucky
The Cancer Capital of the United States

Julie Kiser

CANCER. THIS IS one of the most meaningful and intimidating words I know. When I think of the impact cancer has had on my life, it is daunting to understand the seriousness of this disease. My life has been changed by cancer because of how it has affected my close family. Cancer is prominent in my community, and it affects a large portion of our region. Through faith and determination, we can help the people that suffer from this terrible disease.

My name is Julie Kiser, and I plan to use my future to benefit my community and to contribute to lowering the high incidence of cancer in my region. At Letcher County Central High School, I am learning things in class I hope to use in my future career. In my hometown of Jenkins, Kentucky, I have become keenly aware of cancer and its severity. However, my experiences with cancer have led me to a plan for my future. I was hardly interested in the medical field before I was educated in the science of oncology.

In my future career, I want to go into genetics. I would like to help those who may be affected by mutations in cancer-associated genes. In these situations, there may be something we can do to prevent cancer or lower the risk to the human body. Even if we can't prevent or lower the risk, we can monitor the patients closely to catch the cancer at an early stage. This field of work has interested me ever since I learned that people can be genetically tested for cancer. With the help of genetic testing, I want to help people who could suffer from this disease. I also look forward to helping others who may suffer from other chromosomal disorders and other problems in their hereditary makeup.

My introduction to cancer came when my papaw was diagnosed with multiple myeloma many years ago. Until recently, I had no clue what this meant. Now I understand how multiple myeloma changed so much about him. He couldn't do everything he used to be able to do, and that was difficult for everyone. This type of cancer mainly affected his kidneys, and it metastasized to many of his other organs. One of the main things I remember of my time with him was going with my father to bring him to dialysis. He went every Monday, Wednesday, and Friday for many years. After several years of struggling with this, he passed away, and my family was changed forever. I plan to find out more about multiple myeloma and to begin my own study to understand the causes and how it affects the person suffering from it. I've lost someone important to me without knowing the extensiveness of this disease, and I don't intend to let that happen again.

Cancer also affected a family friend who attends our church. When she was diagnosed with metastatic breast cancer, I knew this could be the reason she could possibly lose her life. I still didn't completely understand the disease when she was diagnosed, but now I understand the full implications of cancer. She was struggling a lot at first. Changing her eating habits was one of the main steps she took to help in her journey of fighting cancer. She went from eating foods like pizza or hot dogs to eating only fruits, vegetables, and some sources of protein. Luckily, she got the help she needed when she was in the early stages of her breast cancer. She underwent chemotherapy for an extended period, leaving her body drained. Despite her struggle for a couple of years, she became cancer free for a while. Tragically, the cancer has returned, this time in her brain. As of now, she is continuing her battle with cancer, and we will pray for her and have hope every step of the way.

From observing my community, I have concluded that Kentucky is greatly affected by smoking and a lack of technology to test for cell mutations that lead to cancer. The main place for people in Kentucky to go is the Markey Cancer Center, but this is a very long travel for some residents. Due to the impact this disease has had on my life, I have taken great interest in it, and I have decided to pursue a career in which I will contribute to helping those diagnosed and to preventing it as much as possible. My main goals, as of now, are to decrease smoking in my community, raise cancer awareness, and provide opportunities to learn about cancer prevention to the people of my community.

I hope to prevent smoking in my community, as I wish I could have done with my papaw. If I were to walk the streets of Jenkins, I'm sure I could see someone smoking a cigarette, and I now understand the damage this is doing to their body. In the future, I want to promote education about the harmful outcomes of smoking. This is such a big issue in my community, and I want that to change. According to the North American Association of Central Cancer Registries, Kentucky has the highest overall cancer incidence and mortality rates in the country in comparison to all other U.S. states.[1] When I learned this, I finally understood how serious the problem in my area truly is. Our daily lifestyle in the Appalachian region is commonly surrounded by harmful habits, like smoking, overexposure to UV rays, and smokeless tobacco, all of which can lead to cancer.

Another reason cancer is so prominent in my community is because there aren't many options open to those in need of screening. Due to this situation, many people can be suffering from any type of cancer and are deprived of the opportunity to understand it. In my area, there are few places to have this testing done. Even with the limited access to screening, there are many people who can't afford to have tests like mammograms or lung cancer scans in the first place. Money is a serious issue in the Appalachian region. For the few who can afford to have cancer screenings done, there is often a significant wait time and/or distance to travel. In many of these instances, people decide it is too much trouble to go through for something they believe to be a cold or a mole.

The new trend of vaping is also harmful to one's body and future. Although it's hard to imagine, many scientists are on their way to proving vaping or e-cigarettes are nearly as bad as smoking real cigarettes. There are many risks involved with these alternatives. The Centers for Disease Control and Prevention (CDC) says that most e-cigarettes contain nicotine, and users are more likely to start smoking cigarettes in the future.[2] This can ultimately lead to a life affected by cancer. There are also multiple harmful carcinogens (cancer-causing substances) that could lead to various forms of cancer. Even after seeing tons of tobacco-prevention commercials, very few people actually realize the truly shocking effects of chewing tobacco, which include gum disease and mouth cancer. This specific type of cancer can also be caused by drinking a lot of alcohol, but tobacco use is much more common than alcohol addiction in my community despite both being serious issues. Apart from my county, there are many parts of Kentucky that have a more severe problem with alcohol addiction. Although there are many attempts to spread awareness of mouth cancer due to tobacco, the number of people using tobacco is only increasing. According to the CDC, the number of middle and high school students using tobacco products increased by 1.3 million between the years 2017 and 2018.[3] Sadly, many of my close friends have taken up the awful habit. Seeing them making this choice has really gotten to me and has caused me to feel passionate about stopping them before it becomes a serious health issue.

Despite all of these causes of cancer in Kentucky, I have many ideas to counteract the high cancer incidence in our state. In my plan, I would start by increasing cancer literacy. We could all try to spread the idea of the seriousness of cancer, and cancer survivors can share their stories as well. Most people never realize the power of words and let the idea of talking about their experiences slip out of their mind. Spreading awareness of cancer encourages those fighting it to continue to follow through with treatments and to never give up. The second step of my plan of addressing cancer in my community is to offer free, planned screenings to those who can't afford to have them done at hospitals. In my county, there are many people financially unable to pay for regular screenings. To be sure of a healthy life free of cancer, it is good to have regular cancer screenings to assure there aren't any tumors. Local hospitals promoting and hosting monthly free screenings could greatly benefit the community, spread awareness, and lower the frequency of cancer in the area. Knowing that the screenings are available will allow some people to discover if they have this life-threatening disease.

Another thing we could do to prevent cancer in Kentucky is to encourage people to be physically active every day. Keeping some exercise in your daily routine prevents many types of cancer. There aren't many ways we could enforce this idea, but there are plenty of ways to encourage it. The National Cancer Institute has studies proving that physical activity can lower the risk of colon, breast, and endometrial cancer.[4] Having free workout programs and multiple recreational centers in the community can support activity among groups of people who don't normally attend recreational centers.

Though there are tons of ways I want to contribute to a better future, I've only mentioned a few. We can improve treatments to make it easier on those who have to endure them and research further into cancer to find more ways to prevent it. In some ways, even those of us who haven't suffered from cancer have still suffered from the ripple effects of seeing our loved ones in pain. When someone we love is hurt by the disease, our lives are altered as well.

Cancer will always be a part of my life and a part of my story. It will always affect the world and the ones we love, no matter how hard we try, but we can do as much as possible to change what we can. If everyone works together to create a better future in Kentucky, we can prevent cancer from becoming more prominent in our state, and we can keep more of our loved ones safe. By spreading knowledge about cancer, we can provide hope to those affected and a better understanding of the seriousness of this disease. By offering all the help we can give, we can provide a better future for the Appalachian region and ultimately cut down the high cancer incidence in our area. This leads to a better future for us and a better life for future generations. Cancer is a scary thing, but if we work together, we can help the world fight it.

Notes

1. North American Association of Central Cancer Registries, "Cancer kills Kentuckians at highest rate (Update)," December 28, 2016, retrieved from https://www.naaccr.org/cancer-kills-kentuckians-at-highest-rate/.

2. Centers for Disease Control and Prevention, "Quick Facts on the Risks of E-cigarettes for Kids, Teens, and Young Adults," retrieved from https://www.cdc.gov/tobacco/basic_information/e-cigarettes/Quick-Facts-on-the-Risks-of-E-cigarettes-for-Kids-Teens-and-Young-Adults.html.

3. Centers for Disease Control and Prevention, "Progress Erased: Youth Tobacco Use Increased During 2017–2018," CDC Online Newsroom, retrieved from https://www.cdc.gov/media/releases/2019/p0211-youth-tobacco-use-increased.html.

4. National Cancer Institute, "Physical Activity and Cancer Fact Sheet," retrieved from https://www.cancer.gov/about-cancer/causes-prevention/risk/obesity/physical-activity-fact-sheet.

The Strength of Family Triumphs All

Kinley Lewis

FAMILY . . . THE REASON for so many of our desires and personal characteristics. Our family and the ones closest to us have such a large impact on our lives and are influential in shaping us into the persons and individuals we strive to be. In my family, we are always one another's "number one fan." We support one another through any situation, and just as we struggle together through any low, we celebrate together during our successes as well.

I am Kinley Lewis, and I am from a small, melancholy town in Elliott County, located in Eastern Appalachian Kentucky. Where I'm from, everyone knows everybody else, and although that can be influential in daily lives, it can also make individual struggles all too real to an entire community. I attend Elliott County High School where I am an upcoming junior. I have ambitions and self-expectations that have led me to the Appalachian Career Training in Oncology (ACTION) Program and opportunities beyond my high school hallways. I am the friend, daughter, and granddaughter of three cancer survivors, all of whom are a huge part of my little family and are the reason for my engagement and aspirations in the medical field and, in particular, the area of oncology.

Being from Elliott County, I consider myself to be the small-town Kentucky girl who has had her share of days walking through fields and fishing by ponds, watching seasons pass from winters with snow that bites through layers, and summers where the sun brings everyone together again. However, we all eventually have to deal with a reality beyond our scenic environment, and that can be much more terrifying than we ever imagined. The colors of our landscape do a more than impressive job of concealing the dangers that we all face and the realities that everyone—no matter their circumstance—will likely come to share. This peril is cancer, the shadow growing behind every corner and over every cliff. Throughout years of research and analysis, the American Cancer Society has concluded that the Appalachian areas of the United States, predominantly Appalachian Kentucky, have a higher percentage of afflicted populations than any other part of the country.[1] Because of this, it is no surprise that my family, like most, has faced multiple hardships in waiting and fighting time and time again to beat the disease that impairs so many. The following are stories about my experiences with cancer.

My Father

My father, John Lewis, was diagnosed with kidney cancer when he was three months old. I can only imagine how my mamaw and papaw—the latter of whom later passed from a benign meningioma—must have felt knowing their child was suffering in a way that they had no way to protect him from. He was diagnosed with a "Wilms' tumor" (nephroblastoma), which is the most common form of childhood kidney cancer; nine out of ten cases of recognized kidney cancer in children are Wilms' tumors.[2] In most cases, including my dad's, the tumor was unilateral, meaning that only one of the two kidneys was affected. When a patient has a bilateral growth, the cancerous cells develop on both kidneys, leading to a higher chance that the cancer will metastasize to other organs. His cancer also had a favorable histology, one in which the cancer cells displayed no signs of anaplasia, making it much easier to treat and remove the tumor safely. Anaplasia occurs when the cells' nuclei are distorted and uneven throughout.[3]

Thankfully, my father's cancer was less severe than it could have been. He was able to have surgery and remove the entirety of the nephroblastoma, followed by chemotherapy and radiation to destroy any remaining abnormal cells. Even though he is cured now, there are still reminders of the effects of his cancer. I can remember when I was younger and just starting to notice details of the things around me, I would ask questions all the time about anything and everything. Granted, I still do that today, just about different things. One summer, when I was probably seven, I was having a pool day with my family, and my dad got in the water with me and my brother. At the time, I was too young to connect the location of the crooked, faded pink, deep scar in his side to something as advanced and beyond my simple-minded imagination as cancer. I would ask and ask question after question about how he got that mark. I needed to know what had happened because all I knew for certain was that I didn't have that on my side, so it must not be normal. Dad used to tell all of us kids that he got it from a shark attack. It was a simple explanation that, knowing my father's joking sense of humor, made perfect sense in the minds of the children he told that to. Although we were all terrified to take a beach trip afterward, we didn't question the scar anymore, and we marveled at the idea of the man who survived the jaws of a great white shark.

My "Second Mom"

When you're from a small town, your friends become family in more ways than you can even imagine. These connections and relationships last life-times through any hardships one might face. There are always constant reassurance and support available to anyone in need in a community like my own. This being said, a very close family friend was diagnosed with cancer almost a year ago. She has always been my "second mom," greeting me with open arms and having an open mind to anything her two children and my brother and I would come up with. Despite the continuous supply of happiness that surrounded our two tightly knit families, we all shared the worry and concern following her diagnosis of stage 2 colorectal cancer. Once the cancer was discovered, there was no time wasted pondering all the "what ifs." She sought doctors who were as prepared and ready as she was in order to fight and survive. The doctors had decided that they would operate and surgically remove the tumor because it was too large to fix simply by using chemo and radiation. However, once they had completed numerous tests and scans, they determined that the tumor was too exten-sive to immediately operate on and that she would have to go through six weeks of chemotherapy in order to shrink the tumor to a size that could be handled surgically. Once those six weeks were over, and the follow-up scans were analyzed, she was scheduled for surgery to remove the cancer and create a stoma (opening) for a colostomy bag to be installed. Origi-nally, the doctors and surgeons believed that they might be able to avoid the need for her to have a colostomy bag. They thought that they would be able to remove the cancer without having to reroute and take out parts of her bowels, but since cancer is wildly unpredictable and ever evolving, the bag was deemed necessary, and that meant another compromise had to be made to ensure all cancerous cells and tissues were properly removed.

After the operation, she had a much deserved and needed period of rest before she had to move on to more preventative measures of twelve more chemo treatments spanning a total of six months. As the end of the months of treatment nears, I realize that the end has been almost harder than the beginning. Most of the worry has begun to cease, but the stress has made faith weak and hearts tired. The last rounds of treatments have been harsher, and each has been followed by a week's worth of side effects. Currently, she has three treatments remaining. By the time this essay is published, she will be finished, and this will all be behind us. If all goes as planned, and if all our prayers have been heard, cancer will once again be defeated, and another life will have been saved.

My Grandfather

One of my closest and longest battles with cancer has been with my grandfather, who has been affected in innumerable ways. My "pap," Billy Waggoner, who is responsible for my random bits of knowledge about planting gardens to feed plenty, working hard for your own sustenance, and the general necessity of having faith in our lives, has gone through three long, hard battles with cancer. Pap worked for years as a tobacco farmer, working in the fields from dawn till dusk with the sun's rays constantly beating down on him. Today, it is common knowledge that everyone needs to apply sunscreen not only to try and keep themselves from getting a sunburn, but also to protect their skin from harmful UVB rays that cause most types of common skin cancers. However, during my pap's working days, sunscreen wasn't a precaution, and after years of prolonged unprotected exposure to the sun, he has had multiple skin cancers of varying sizes and severities.

The first of his battles began in 1997, six years before I was born. He was diagnosed with squamous cell carcinoma originally located on his gum, but it had metastasized to his neck. The doctors described his tumor as being about the size of a lemon. After the discovery, he began a treatment plan consisting of radiation therapy every day for eight weeks to try and shrink the tumor to a size that could be surgically removed. Once that course ended, more scans were performed, and upon their analysis the doctors concluded that the radiation had done more than originally hoped. It had not only reduced the size of the tumor, but it had also completely irradiated the cancer from his gum—meaning that the surgery would no longer be as extensive as they had previously planned. They scheduled his operation, and his surgeons were able to remove the entire mass from his neck, leaving him cancer free for almost fifteen years.

In 2012, I was in second grade. I had just moved to a new elementary school and can remember making all kinds of new friends and the fun we had playing outside at recess. Around the middle of the school year, my pap was diagnosed with a second squamous cell carcinoma—this time in his ear canal. Once again, he went to the Markey Cancer Center for more scans and labs. The doctors said that the newly found cancer that had been growing in his ear canal had quickly spread to his temporal bone and the upper layers of his dura. The dura matter consists of three membrane layers known as meninges that surround the brain and spinal cord, providing protection for the central nervous system.[4] The doctors immediately began preparing for treatment and surgery. I can remember it being very stressful for me, and I really couldn't comprehend all the organized chaos going on around me, much less how my pap and my mother must have felt.

When his medical care first began, the doctors started with a radical neck dissection. They removed the tumor from his ear canal, but in the process, they had to make the necessary call to sever the jugular vein because the tumor was growing around it. They rerouted the vein to the other side of his neck to keep it functional. After this surgery was completed, he underwent a second operation of a temporal bone resection. Here, they removed the cancer from his head and separated two layers of the upper dura from the brain: the dura matter and the arachnoid matter. They believed this eliminated most of the cancerous cells, but in order to be sure no cancer remained, he had six weeks of chemotherapy and radiation. His radiation was daily, and he had chemo on a weekly basis. Now, for a second time, we believed that he was cancer free.

That idea ended two years ago in 2017 when, for a third time, pap was diagnosed with cancer, this time a brain tumor that was believed to have begun as a growth as a result of remaining cells from his previous cancer. He was tired; he had already fought longer and harder than any one person should ever have to fight. He had already spent years in hospitals and going to doctor's appointments. This time we thought that he had taken all he could bear, that there just wasn't enough strength to push with this time, until one of his doctors had a new proposition. He said that pap's cancer was too small to surgically remove, that more damage would be caused if they tried to do an operation. Naturally, we believed it was a good thing, and it was. The mass was only the size of a fingertip, but later we realized that if we didn't do anything that the tumor would only be left to grow. If that happened, we would have an even bigger problem to try and fix later, whether that be months or years down the road. With this thought in mind, his doctors came to us with a new therapy known as a gamma knife treatment.

Gamma knife radiosurgery, a type of stereotactic radiosurgery, does not use incisions. Instead, during a gamma knife treatment, the specialist uses two hundred microbeams of radiation pinpointed on a single focal point, the tumor, to expose it to high doses of radiation while leaving minimal damage to surrounding healthy brain tissue. In most cases, a gamma knife treatment is a one-time-only therapy and is typically completed in one day.[5] This makes it easier for patients like my pap, who are no longer able to go through major surgery and weeks of recovery, to still be able to seek treatment. Gamma knife treatment doesn't necessarily rid a patient of a tumor or mass, but it does stunt its growth and its cells' replication. This means that although the problem doesn't go away, it is very likely that it does not get worse. For smaller, less severe cases, gamma knife treatment is an amazing tool for oncologists to utilize. Based on this information, my pap went home, and after deliberating his options and weighing his pros and cons, he decided to do the gamma knife. The relief we felt after this decision was surreal. We knew now that maybe he could win this battle too, that he could live again and continue to be my fighter and inspiration.

Currently, two years after his gamma knife treatment, my pap goes to the hospital every six months for an MRI. His doctors are always looking for new growth or any signs of change to his tumor. Thankfully, there has been no recurrent growth. His brain tumor is still only the size of a fingertip, and based on his last scan, the doctor said that if anything, the growth had only shrunk. To me, the miracles medicine holds and its abilities to change lives are incredible. After three long hard battles, my pap is still with us. He's a little hard of hearing, but he's still the same fighter he was back in 1997 and is by far the strongest man I know. He will always be my main inspiration to work for the things I want, and he will always be the motivation behind any and all of my medical ambitions. I can only hope to be able to push through what he did with my future patients. I want to be the reason someone else gets to live again too.

Solutions

As I stated earlier, Kentucky has the highest rates of cancer incidence and mortality than any other state in the United States. That can partially correspond with the large population of individuals that abuse cancer-causing substances such as tobacco. Our area also has poor health standards when it comes to diet, and obesity carries multiple health risks including cancer. Since I have been accepted into the ACTION Program, I have been educating my family and friends about Kentucky's high rates of cancer. I am repeatedly stunned by the fact that the majority of people I have spoken to do not know that Kentucky has the highest cancer rates of all states. I have found many adults I know aren't fully aware of the dangers of cancer or how to prevent it. According to the American Cancer Society, since 2015 lung and bronchus cancer has consistently been one of the top five most common cancer types nationally and the top cancer type in our state.[6] If you look at the characteristics of people in our region, a prominent statistic is the number of people who smoke and use tobacco. Although smoking rates are decreasing overall, it is still very prominent in Appalachian areas.

Another characteristic of the people in our state that contributes to the high cancer rates is diet. People are not consuming the right foods. Many individuals regularly ingest overly processed foods, whether that be through frozen meals or packaged snack items. The preservatives and low nutritional values of processed foods are a large contributor to the growing number of obese and overweight people in our communities. It is common knowledge that being overweight can cause health issues such as high blood pressure, higher risk of stroke, type 2 diabetes, and other cardiovascular diseases. Most people, however, are unaware that being obese also increases the likelihood that they could be diagnosed with cancer. Increased weight gain can contribute to cancer because fat cells can alter processes that affect cancer cell growth factors. If there are chronic levels of inflammation in an individual due to the increase in fat, their adipokine levels and certain signaling processes within the body can be altered, leading to an increased risk of cancer development.[7] A person with type 2 diabetes is at an increased risk as well, because high levels of insulin have been linked to cancer.

Finally, one of Kentucky's main issues is the ineffective or nonexistent health education of our state's population, primarily minors. If we could more effectively teach our communities about the risk factors associated with cancer, people might be more inclined to change their routines in order to lessen their chances of developing this disease. Our children need to hear about cancer risk factors, such as obesity and smoking, for more than one day at a single school event. Providing information one time will not solve the problem; the key to ending this issue is consistent and repeated teaching. It would help to remind people of things they can do to protect themselves so that they might avoid having to go through battles like my pap did. More efforts are needed to decrease tobacco abuse and to promote having a healthy diet or, if possible, simply eating fewer processed foods. Since we live in a beautiful area surrounded by nature, we all need to apply sunscreen to protect our skin. Sometimes, simple adjustments in our daily lives can go a long way toward preventing cancer.

When we think of curing cancer, people tend to imagine a miracle drug. However, instead of having such a definite and limiting idea, we need to realize that cancer can be defeated by something as simple and easy as putting sunscreen on our face.

Conclusion

Through the ACTION Program, I am one of twenty high school students who are getting the chance to put my hand in on the war against cancer. We all share experiences, like my own, with family members or friends who have suffered because of cancer. Every person involved in making this program possible has one common goal in mind: to bring new minds and more ideas to the table in order for more progress to be made against cancer. I'm in this fight for my dad, for my friend, and for my pap, the three strongest people I know. As a student still impressionable to the world around me, I'm constantly debating new ideas about everything imaginable, which is why we need young minds on the task of thinking in ways previously unknown in medicine. In ACTION, we are the future. We are the teens and the students and the individuals who will eventually have a say in future medical history. I cannot wait to see what we accomplish.

Notes

1. American Cancer Society, "2018 Cancer Facts & Statistics: Kentucky at a glance," retrieved June 22, 2019, from https://cancerstatisticscenter.cancer.org/#!/state/Kentucky.

2. American Cancer Society, "What Are Wilms Tumors?" 2018, retrieved June 22, 2019, from https://www.cancer.org/cancer/wilms-tumor/about/what-is-wilms-tumor.html.

3. Ibid.

4. National Cancer Institute, "Definition of Dura Mater," retrieved July 23, 2019, from https://www.cancer.gov/publications/dictionaries/cancer-terms/def/dura-mater.

5. https://www.mayoclinic.org/tests-procedures/brain-stereotactic-radiosurgery/about/pac-20384679.

6. American Cancer Society, "2018 Cancer Facts & Statistics: Kentucky at a glance," retrieved June 22, 2019, from https://cancerstatisticscenter.cancer.org/#!/state/Kentucky.

7. https://www.cancer.gov/about-cancer/causes-prevention/risk/obesity/obesity-fact-sheet#what-is-known-about-the-relationship-between-obesity-and-cancer-.

The Greatest Ideas Are the Simplest
Educating Kentuckians on Cancer

Nolan Marcum

MOST PEOPLE KNOW me as Nolan Isaiah Marcum, and I am a determined teenager with a big dream. Most of my friends call me W.I.N., because if you flip my initials upside down and backward, they spell WIN. I am from Carter County, Kentucky, and have lived there my entire life. My hometown of Grayson is a very small community within Carter County, and there isn't anything to do there besides bowling. Grayson is a town where everyone knows one another, which means I can have better relationships with my teachers and friends, and that is a spectacular opportunity. I am in the class of 2021 at East Carter High School and tied for first place in my graduating class with an unweighted GPA of 4.0. I participate in several extracurricular activities and programs. For example, Beta Club allows me to be intertwined with my hometown through community service opportunities. Another great activity is Unified Club, through which we assist special-needs children, giving them a chance at playing sports and games and attending community-service activities.

Similar to many of my ACTION (Appalachian Career Training in Oncology) Program classmates, I have put a lot of thought into what I would like to pursue as a career. Since I was young, I have known that I want to be a forensic scientist. Plans usually change as you become older, but not much for me. I knew that I loved forensics, watching anatomical procedures and learning about anatomy. I ultimately have chosen a career that combines all of my interests: a forensic pathologist. My family isn't really crazy about my dream of becoming a forensic pathologist. Although they are supportive, they don't understand why I would want to stare at dead bodies all day.

Additionally, I absolutely love my advanced placement biology class. I enjoy learning everything about cells' functions, tissues, and how the body responds to and repairs injury. I have the best teacher in the state of Kentucky teaching my class, Mrs. Bonzo. Mrs. Bonzo has helped me a lot this year. I know I can be hard to handle because I ask many hard questions when I get excited, but she has strengthened my love for science. As I mentioned earlier, I enjoy anatomy. One of my goals is to perform a real-life autopsy on a cadaver, just to see what it's like.

Outside of forensics, I really enjoy studying and researching cancer. Oncology is such an open and interesting field, stretching throughout all branches of medicine. The cancers I find most interesting are hormonal cancers. The reason I favor hormonal cancers is because I enjoy the endocrine system's complexity and the intricacies of all the hormone pathways. There is a great amount to learn about the endocrine system, especially when you throw something like cancer, with all its mutations, at it.

I am actually closely affected by cancer because of my mother. When I was a young kid, my parents were addicted to drugs. I've watched my mother pass out because she has overdosed countless times. After watching my mother overdose, I knew that I wanted to do something meaningful with my life, instead of being a drug addict. I wanted to achieve great things and maybe one day help my mother—hopefully, if she is still living. My father wasn't as fortunate as she has been, so I don't have the opportunity to save him. I blame myself because if I had the knowledge of how to treat drug addiction before he overdosed, maybe I could have saved his life. My mother is still addicted to drugs despite my father's tragedy and countless other tragedies that she has witnessed.

A few years ago, my mother was diagnosed with bladder cancer. She absolutely refused chemotherapy for the longest time. It was extremely hard to watch my mom look like a zombie. She was always tired and very sick. Since my mother didn't go to her treatments as I insisted, she turned to self-medicating, which my family didn't take very well. We all love her so much, but none of us said anything at the time. This was where the blame falls on me. I'm the second youngest sibling out of the four. I'm the most responsible, so I should have been the one to handle this. My sister was having a rough time handling the situation for about the first month of the news. I helped her through it as much as possible. I thank the Lord for the book *Lord of the Flies* because it helped me relate what was happening in my life to what was happening to the boys on the island. They had to govern themselves, and they split apart from one another as time went on. With my mother in the situation she was, I had to basically take care of myself and my younger sister. My older brothers would always be off somewhere doing what they wanted with their friends and were almost never home. Every time I read the book, I would find more to relate to. I read that book probably at least five times a week. My time was occupied predominantly by two things: football and *The Lord of the Flies*. If I hadn't had these activities, I don't think I would have made it without breaking down as my sister did every week. As time went on, the house became even more gloomy. To make matters worse, I didn't agree with my mother's choices, and my mother wasn't taking the diagnosis very well, so she acted out. I'm not sure I can blame her for this—I can't say what I would have done if the doctor had given me only six months to live. For three months, she refused to get any treatments. I prayed every night that she would eventually come to her senses and do the right thing, not for me, but for my sister. I just couldn't stand watching my sister being ripped apart over this anymore. After a long talk, thankfully she came to her senses. She has also been to rehab to get back on the right track. Now my mother has been going to her treatments for about a year or so. It isn't all rainbows and sunshine. My mother still has bladder cancer, and it can be a hard thing to think about some days. Other days it can be embarrassing when we are in public, but overall my family is in a lot better shape than what it was. Thankfully, through her radiation treatments, she has been able to fight back against the horrific bladder cancer. My mother is my closest cancer-related incident, but not my only one. Several family members and many of my friends' families have had cancer.

Although my situation is rather unfortunate, it isn't rare to any of us who live here in Appalachian Kentucky. Sadly, it's rather normal. According to the Northern American Association of Central Cancer Registries (NAACCR), Eastern Kentucky has the highest incidence rates for cancer. Unfortunately, we are also ranked number one in the United States for the highest cancer mortality rates.[1] Furthermore, we have the greatest population that is diagnosed with several types of cancer, and we far exceed the national average in lung and bronchus cancer.[2]

Unsurprisingly, the main cause of cancer deaths in Kentucky is tobacco. It isn't a coincidence that Kentucky leads America in the highest diagnosed cancer population. We also have the highest rate of cancer deaths caused by tobacco use, according to the Centers for Disease Control and Prevention (CDC).[3] The CDC also documents that Kentucky is ranked second in the number of smokers in the United States, just barely under West Virginia. I would without a doubt say smoking tobacco plays the largest role in why Kentuckians are developing cancer more often than people in other states.

I have a personal story about tobacco causing cancer. I couldn't say that tobacco is the largest contributor of cancer and expect people to believe what I say if I didn't have a personal experience with evidence to let people truly understand my perspective. My uncle was also diagnosed with lung cancer. I will be the first one to tell you that my uncle would smoke more than the average person in Kentucky. Of course, my siblings and I would always tell him that he was going to end up regretting the choice one day. My uncle was a stubborn old man, and he never did quit. Sadly, stubbornness over the addiction to nicotine did cause my uncle's death. This is the story of how my uncle battled against tobacco use and its horrific side effects.

Cigarettes aren't the only reason our cancer incidence and mortality rates are higher than anywhere else. I believe it's also occurring in Kentucky because, compared to other states, we have a relatively low education level. According to US News, Kentucky is ranked thirty-eighth in the United States for overall education. From kindergarten to twelfth-grade education, Kentucky is ranked thirty-second.[4]

I would debate that being an undereducated population is the second-worst epidemic Kentucky faces, almost as bad as our cancer epidemic. Poverty rates may be the first thing that you might think of when it comes to low education level. Less-educated people will have an increased probability of having lower-income jobs.[5] If most of the population has lower-income jobs, it's harder for adults to afford healthcare. This can result in a certain number of people who will not obtain the checkups they should get. This can lead to the growth of a tumor over a long period that might have been easily removed, but the tumor was not detected in time, so it became deadly. According to "Society Health," lower-educated populations tend to be less aware of their environment, thus causing them not to care about what is going on in their communities.[6] I believe most Kentuckians don't take care of the environment. This can lead to a variety of issues, such as metals in the water like arsenic, copper, and lead. This process is called acid mine drainage.[7]

Additionally, Kentucky is also undereducated about the contents of tobacco products. The majority of Kentucky really doesn't have a grasp on the harmful facts. Although the majority know smoking kills us, that is not enough. If it were, no one would be smoking. What smokers don't know is that it is the toxins in cigarettes that put the strain and toll on their bodies.

I believe Kentuckians are smarter than people give us credit for. We are not imbeciles who are just mindlessly smoking for no reason. Most older smokers came from generations that weren't well educated about cigarettes. During the mid-1900s, smoking started getting very popular. Everyone did it, without fully knowing the side effects such as cancer. Most of our parents started smoking at a young age and became addicted to cigarettes. That is why smoking became such an epidemic. Everyone got hooked on it before we could learn what was really in cigarettes, like arsenic, methanol, and methane. These harmful ingredients are what I feel most people who smoke didn't spend time to learn or care about. Maybe some of our parents know, but children don't know the damage it's doing to their close loved ones.

Lung and bronchus cancer is the most common cancer in Kentucky, and it is often caused by smoking.[8] We need to try to slow down the rate of these cancers primarily. I believe the best course of action to address the cancer epidemic in Kentucky is to really start where the greatest harm is: lung cancer. The way to do this is to educate the younger population more about cancer: what cancer is, and how it's affecting Kentucky. If we educate more minds about how harmful cancer can be, there is a greater chance they will avoid environments that are more prone to cancer, such as being around people who tend to be smokers. Staying away from these types of environments will lower the cancer incidence rates.[9] Along with that, we can address the cancer epidemic by educating the younger population on a topic that is widely known by all Kentuckians: smoking! We can inform young adults of the harmful ingredients in tobacco products and how they can cause life-threatening cancers in their parents, loved ones, or even themselves. It's essential for Kentuckians to comprehend the atrociousness of tobacco that is never advertised. Furthermore, we can educate people on how these chemicals will affect your body and show them the effects that smoking has on their body. For example, as *Physician's Weekly* states, smoking can damage aspects of vision.[10] By educating them on this topic, I hope it will put fear into them not only for themselves, but for their close relatives and friends. It will act like dominoes, thus lowering the smoking rates for future generations. Furthermore, these children can go to their parents and close loved ones and teach them what they are putting in their bodies. The children would want their parents to abandon these horrific habits, knowing that smoking causes cancer. The American Cancer Society states that nicotine is highly addictive and is absorbed easily into the blood thereby allowing it to spread through the entire body. Men and women who use tobacco are usually heavily addicted to tobacco, and it's very challenging to fight addiction alone.[11] My hopes for teaching younger children about smoking is that they will want to help their loved ones fight it together. Hopefully, if an adult knows children want them to quit, they eventually will quit smoking.

So, I believe that the most efficient way to address the cancer epidemic is to clearly educate the younger population more about the terrible chemicals in cigarettes and to decrease smoking rates, which will eventually also decrease cancer rates.

Notes

1. Charlie Blackburn, "Cancer kills Kentuckians at highest rate," 2016, https://www.naaccr.org/cancer-kills-kentuckians-at-highest-rate/.

2. NCI, Cancer Statistics, https://www.cancer.gov/about-cancer/understanding/statistics.

3. "CDC Newsroom," 2016, https://www.cdc.gov/tobacco/data_statistics/state_data/state_highlights/2012/states/kentucky/index.htm.

4. "These U.S. States Have the Best Education Systems," Usnews.com, n.d., https://www.usnews.com/news/best-states/rankings.

5. "How does the level of education relate to poverty?" 2015, https://poverty.ucdavis.edu/faq/how-does-level-education-relate-poverty.

6. "Why education matters to health: Exploring the causes," 2015, https://societyhealth.vcu.edu/work/the-projects/why-education-matters-to-health-exploring-the-causes.html.

7. The Union of Concerned Scientists, "Coal and water pollution," 2017, https://www.ucsusa.org/clean-energy/coal-and-other-fossil-fuels/coal-water-pollution.

8. NCI, Cancer Statistics, https://www.cancer.gov/about-cancer/understanding/statistics.

9. "Cancer Epidemiology and Cancer Prevention," n.d., https://www.hsph.harvard.edu/cecp/student-spotlight/.

10. Linda Carroll, "Chemical in cigarette smoke may damage important aspect of vision," 2018, https://www.physiciansweekly.com/chemical-in-cigarette-smoke/.

11. The American Cancer Society medical and editorial content team, "Why People Start Using Tobacco, and Why It's Hard to Stop," 2015, https://www.cancer.org/cancer/cancer-causes/tobacco-and-cancer/why-people-start-using-tobacco.html.

Tales into Legacies

Alyviah Newby

NOTHING IS MORE precious than the relationship between a grandfather and his granddaughter or a father and his little girl. These are not tales, but legacies of the ones who fought for life and a second chance. Eleanor Roosevelt once said, "You gain strength, courage, and confidence by every experience in which you really stop to look fear in the face. You must do the thing which you think you cannot do." These are the legacies of my grandpa and uncle.

I'm Alyviah Newby, and I am from Russell County, Kentucky. I'm a rising sophomore at Russell County High School, the home of the Lakers. If there is one topic with which we can all relate in my county, it is the effects of cancer on the ones whom we hold near and dear. Growing up, I was raised in a big family. The silent killer we call cancer has been flowing through generations of the blood of my family members.

I was just eight years old when I told my world, my best friend, the one I call grandpa, goodbye. He was the best grandpa that I could've asked for, but it was unfortunate that he wasn't a big part of my life until he found out that he had stage 4 non-Hodgkin's lymphoma and moved to Kentucky for his final resting place. During the year of his sufferings, I never noticed how weak and pale he was getting. He never wanted my sister and me to see him at his lowest time of this battle that he was fighting. When he came to Kentucky, it was summer break for my sister and me, and he slept on the couch at my house for a few weeks. In those few weeks, I slept on the couch with him. My parents eventually got him a house right up the road from ours, and every morning when I woke up, I rushed to put my shoes on (and sometimes I didn't even put on shoes!) because I tried to spend every minute with him, playing and spending quality time with him. One day, my parents allowed my grandpa to watch my sister and me so they could run some errands. They left, and at this time my sister and I thought it was a great idea to get grandpa's wheelchair and ride it down the hill that was on the road. When we asked my grandpa, he said, "Ok, just don't hurt yourselves," then my parents came back and saw my sister and me on a wheelchair going down the hill. At first, they were laughing, but then they told us to stop. When they went inside and asked my grandpa why we were on the wheelchair, he said, "They are kids. Let them have fun." He was with us for his birthday, my sister's birthday, my birthday, and Thanksgiving. Sadly, he passed away in his sleep on December 22, 2011. It was peaceful, and he wasn't suffering anymore. For Christmas, my mom and dad got him a wallet that he wanted. Every year, we leave his wrapped present under the tree first and pack it up last. Even though I miss him very deeply, I know that one day I will see him again.

I have a lot of cousins, and it's pretty crazy when the most unexpected thing happens to them. My cousin Addacin was just eight years old when her dad was diagnosed with stage 3 glioblastoma. He was the world to her. They had a bond that nobody could separate, but cancer did. Cancer took her world, the one whom she called Superman, the one who was supposed to walk her down the aisle and give her away at her wedding. It became surgery after surgery for the last two years until November 2017. Addacin was getting ready for school and noticed that her dad, Jordan, was acting stranger than usual. By this time, he had had so many seizures he was paralyzed on his entire left side, and he had his toilet and hospital bed in the living room of their house. He couldn't be by himself for five minutes without trying to walk and be independent. My aunt Beckie had to turn to hospice because she needed extra help in taking care of him. While Addacin was at school, the workers in the office called her up so she could leave without knowing that she had to face the ending of her and her father's relationship together. They arrived at the hospital, and she thought that Jordan was just having a spell. She thought the hospital would fix it and they could go home, but that wasn't the case. The doctors gave him two days to live. Addacin's heart broke into pieces, and she didn't leave his side. She lay there on the hospital bed next to him.

I received a text message that same day from my aunt Bonnie, saying, "Pray for Jordan. They are giving him a day or two to live." I was on the school bus when I read it, and I just started crying. Many people didn't know how to react to my crying because they had never seen me cry as I did that evening. As soon as I got off the bus, I rushed down the road to my house to see if my mom was there, but she was already at the hospital. My dad was home, and I asked if I could go to the hospital, but my dad didn't want me to see Jordan in that condition.

It was a Wednesday night; he had already passed the date that the doctors had expected him to live, and my church decided to bring kids to the hospital to sing to him. I couldn't lay my eyes on him because seeing him groaning in pain and asking for water was nearly too much to handle. When it was my turn to sing, I couldn't hit a single note without crying. Several days passed, and Jordan was a trooper. When Friday came, Beckie had to leave the hospital to get something to eat because she couldn't bear to eat one more plate of hospital food. When she left, it was just my mom and I. He was slowly dying at this point; every ten minutes one of us had to press the button so he could get more morphine to take some pain away. He was wearing an oxygen mask because he wasn't getting enough air on his own. His skin was discolored, and his urine was burnt orange in color because his kidneys were shutting down. Addacin's little brother, Nolan, gave Jordan a stuffed dog that was singing "Jesus Loves Me." Jordan was mumbling along with it, so I sat down next to him. I was holding his hand on his right side so he would know that someone was there for him, and I began to sing to him. After the dog stopped singing, I began to sing hymns and choir songs. As I was singing to him, one of the nurses came in to change his fluids and upped his morphine and said, "You have a beautiful voice. I bet he is enjoying it." I replied, "I'm pretty sure he is." She looked at him and patted his foot, saying, "People can't say the cancer won if they didn't see them fighting it." I will never forget what she said that night. It was Saturday night, and at this point, Addacin didn't want to leave because she wanted to be there to tell him goodbye. Every day that week, Addacin would walk out of the hospital with tears streaming down her face, but on Saturday night, I was holding her in my arms. She melted on my shoulder when she had to leave.

I remember Sunday, the day that he died, so vividly. I was at church and singing "Farther Along," one of my favorite hymns. As we were singing, my friend Lisa told me that Bonnie was in the back and had to tell me something. When I headed back there, she told me that they were going to give Jordan medicine that would allow him to pass. Luckily, the church was right across from the hospital. I got to the hospital and went down the wing to his room. My uncle Aaron and Bonnie were only letting two people go into the room at a time to say their goodbyes. Finally, it was time for my mom and me to say goodbye. The room was dark when I entered, and it had cooled down since it wasn't crowded. At this point, he was so discolored you couldn't tell if he was human, and if you could, you wouldn't know if he was alive or not. Beckie was in a chair right next to him, holding his hand through the whole passing. My goodbye was formal. I grabbed his hand tightly. The hand that I held as my way of saying goodbye had some feeling to it, but to me, it was just another dead part of his body. It was hot, clammy, and purple. When I walked out of the room, my face was white as a ghost. When we got to the car, my mom told me not to set foot on the hospital's property because she didn't want me to witness his death. So I walked back to the church, and I was there for two hours. In those two hours, I was thinking about Jordan. When I got in my mom's car, church was over. I didn't have to ask because I already knew by mom's facial expression that he was gone.

That night, Addacin was staying the night at our grandma's house, and our grandma told Addacin that he had passed. I was shocked at how she reacted; I didn't think she would take it as easily as she did. After his funeral, I remember seeing that Addacin was so happy—like nothing had happened and everything was normal. I think she was happy because she knew that Jordan would want her to be happy.

Ever since those two personal encounters, I have always had a strange fascination with cancer. I have wanted to be a neurosurgeon like Ben Carson. I want to do something to end the war of cancer among the millions of people suffering. I want to find a cure or just something that will give people who have been affected by this turmoil a longer time to live and be with their families and loved ones. Sometimes, I feel that we take life for granted even though our lives are nothing but vapor.

I believe there is a way to reduce the high rate of cancer in Kentucky. I believe it would help reduce cancer in Kentucky if we implement health awareness for kids, teens, and adults about the benefits of living a healthy lifestyle and making good choices. Not only that, but if we reduce the rate of smoking, there will be a drastic improvement to the smokers themselves, the surrounding people, and the environment. It's sad to say that I live in a state with the highest percentage of cancer. According to the North American Association of Central Cancer Registries, "Kentucky has the highest overall cancer incidence and mortality in the country compared to all other U.S states and the District of Columbia."[1] I think the reason why cancer affects Kentuckians so badly is because of bad habits and poor decisions. I also think we need to spend more time in spreading awareness to people in our communities about cancer and its deadly effect on us as well as future generations.

One day, hopefully, there will be a cure for this killer so that it cannot take more precious lives of people around us, and Kentucky's cancer incidence can decrease. When that day comes, we won't have to worry about treatments or the chance of survival anymore.

Notes

1. C. Blackburn, *Cancer Kills Kentuckians At Highest Rate (Update)*, March 28, 2016, retrieved from North American Association of Central Cancer Registries: www.naaccr.org/cancer-kills-kentuckians-at-highest-rate/.

Ripped at the Seams

Katelyn Nigro

CANCER, THE WORD that no one likes to hear or say, the word that puts a knot in your stomach, the word that makes your heart break for those who are or have been victims. Cancer is an aggressive and dangerous disease that, in 2019, is predicted to have 1,762,450 new cases in the United States.[1] Kentucky is unfortunately the most affected state in America.[2] There are many things that could affect these cancer rates; I believe that Kentucky's rates are linked to smoking, obesity, coal dust, and the lack of opportunity for preventative screenings. Kentucky is a rural southern state that many call home but also where many fall prey to cancer. My goal is to spread awareness about the risk factors and make screenings obtainable for those in my region. My name is Katelyn Nigro; I live in Corbin, Kentucky, and this is my experience with cancer.

Our grandparents are the glue that holds a family together. They keep family dinners and holidays consistent. They are the best storytellers, best cooks, and often like a second set of parents. My paternal grandparents both fell victim to lung cancer, and it has taken a toll on my family. I have very little memory of my grandmother because I was so young when she passed. I only really know what my parents have told me about her. In fact, the only thing I can recall is her voice. My younger brother doesn't even have that. In November 2006, my grandmother was diagnosed with stage 4 small-cell lung cancer, and she was given six to eight months to live. Hard and trying months passed by with no improvement. When she knew the inevitable was coming, my grandmother decided to go above and beyond for her last Christmas. She bought extravagant Christmas presents for everyone such as expensive watches and collectible items because she wanted to be remembered, and she is indeed in all of our hearts. For her last six months my grandmother lived with my aunt, and while living there, she would help watch me while my parents worked. My grandmother's whole life was her grandchildren. One of her many dreams was to build a lake house in Tennessee with a dock and boat for her family to enjoy. My grandfather started to build her dream house, but unfortunately, she never got to see it. My grandmother passed away in May 2007, almost six months after her diagnosis. Tragically, she was only fifty-two when she left this world. When she passed, she left me her gold jewelry that I have kept locked away for years for fear of losing it. I wear the locket she left me for good luck on special occasions. I wear it on church holidays and every time I take the ACT; I wore it to my first job interview, and most recently, I wore it to take my driver's test. I wear it so that I know she's there with me. When I was younger, she gave me a white and brown stuffed dog that I cherished deeply. I used to refuse to sleep without it. Now, I keep it in my closet as a reminder of her. Cancer robbed me of memories with my grandmother and robbed her of a life with her grandchildren.

My life continued normally for about five years, but then it was flipped entirely upside down. In April 2012, my paternal grandfather was diagnosed with stage 4 small-cell lung cancer. This was a moment of shock for my family. Our whole world stopped turning and came crashing down around us. Fortunately, the doctors were able to do a partial lobectomy and completely remove the cancer. My family rejoiced. We dreaded losing him the same way we had my grandmother. In August 2013, the cancer was back. It had returned, and this time was stronger than before. My grandfather fought hard through his treatments, only becoming weaker and weaker. I had no memory of grandmother's journey, but I remember everything about his. In October 2013, we made a huge decision. We decided to move my grandfather from Lake City, Tennessee, into our house in Corbin, Kentucky. I remember watching his decline daily. His skin became paler, his waist thinner, his muscles weaker. His mind started slipping, and I watched it all happen. For his last Christmas with us, he took our entire family to Disney World—a nearly $15,000 trip dedicated to us and the memories he wanted us to have. When I look back at the pictures, I see how sick he looked. I see how serious this disease that I didn't know much about really was. With him living at our home, I had to learn how to help with many of his treatment routines and his care. I did other things that didn't have to do with medical care. I made him coffee every morning and washed his clothes, and I'd even make his oatmeal. I did anything I could to help my parents care for him. Time passed, and he soon started having to use oxygen around the clock. He got so weak he had to use a walker, and he started seeing things that weren't there. Soon we began realizing that the end of his fight was coming. In February 2014, I lost my grandfather. I remember every day prior to his passing clearly. Every day when I got picked up from school, I asked how he was and waited for the dreaded response, but I never got it. Until one day, I had spent the day at my uncle's house with my cousins and we got the call. My parents didn't want me to have to see him in his bed, but as I walked by to my room for an overnight bag, I saw him, and I'll never forget it. It was surreal that he was really gone. That was the first time I had ever really experienced death.

Cancer affected not only my grandparent's lives but also all of the lives around them. The cancer caused our family dynamic to change. It caused financial and emotional stress and decline. When my grandmother was put in the hospital, we knew that the outcome wasn't promising as the results of the biopsy had returned in less than an hour. So my grandfather rushed to fulfill the dream of a lake house that she wanted. He had to use so much money for that house and her care.

My grandmother lived with my aunt during her treatment, and during her time there she received home hospice care. Hospice care for my grandmother consisted of a nurse who would come to the house a few days a week and check on how she was doing. In my experience, hospice is a huge relief, but also a bit of a hindrance. You have to alter your schedule to be home when the nurse will be there and such. When my grandmother died, it drove wedges between the family, causing major problems. It had a huge impact on my father and on his sister, and my father is still affected by it today. My grandmother's death started a grudge between my father and his sister—one that would only grow. My family was being ripped apart piece by piece.

Both of my paternal grandparents were heavy smokers, and so when my grandfather was diagnosed with stage 4 lung cancer, it was no surprise. He had been getting spontaneous fractures in his spine and pneumonia very frequently. We saw my grandfather weekly. We'd go to his house in Tennessee and play cards with him and his girlfriend. We loved sliding cards under the table to mess with him. Then, things took a turn for the worse, so we moved him to Kentucky with us. It forced me and my brother to share a room, and that didn't help ease any sibling bickering. We had to introduce our grandfather's dog to our dogs, and that was a literal dog fight. We rebuilt parts of our house for him so that things would be easier to access. It took a toll on our family and how we ran our household. We would wake up to hear him coughing at night, or he would get something in his mind, and we would have to calm him back into bed. I remember one scary night when we thought the worst was coming. It didn't though, and my dad was trying to get him to stay awake, but also needed to go get medicine to help. I jumped in to help; I kept him awake by telling him one of his favorite shows was on, *Judge Judy,* and also by talking about politics. Politics really brought the loud Italian out in him. After my grandfather's death is when the divide of my family really came. Things came up in the will that caused a great upset in the family. Now, my father and his sister haven't spoken in about five years. My father lost both of his parents by the age of forty-five, and it was extremely hard on him. Every Mother's Day, Father's Day, and Grandparent's Day, I see the look of grief on my father's face.

Aside from the emotional impact our loss had on everyone in the family, cancer has also imposed a constant feeling of fear in me. Like his parents, my father is a smoker, and smoking can lead to cancer. Over the years, my father has tried to quit smoking many times. He has tried many methods, yet somehow he always starts again. I love my father dearly, and the last thing I want is for cancer to tear him away from his family, as it did my grandparents. My father is one of my biggest supporters, and I want to help fight anything that puts him at risk.

I want to help to prevent cancer in the state of Kentucky. I want to help make people aware of the risks that exist in our beautiful home. Obviously, tobacco is a huge issue. In Kentucky, 24.6 percent of adults are smokers.[3] This major carcinogen can lead to lung cancer and mouth cancer, as reported by The Oral Cancer Foundation and American Lung Association. I believe that the rate of teen and even adult users is likely to increase unless people are educated about the many harmful risks. Another huge problem is obesity and an overweight population. Obese people often have chronic low-level inflammation, and inflammation can cause DNA damage and the overproduction of certain chemicals in the body, which could lead to cancer.[4] Another reason why I consider Kentucky the cancer state is because of coal mining in our state through many generations. As discussed earlier, Kentucky has a high rate of smokers. Many men who have worked in the coal mines in Kentucky most likely picked up the habit while working in the mines. During their careers, they also could have inhaled coal dust, which can lead to pneumoconiosis, or "black lung." Pneumoconiosis causes scarring in the lungs and creates inflammation that can make lung cancer easier to contract when both pneumoconiosis and a smoking addiction are present.[5] Lastly, there is a lack of ability to get regular cancer screenings and education. Kentucky has a poor rural southeastern region where many people don't have the means to pay for cancer screenings. Because of this, when or if cancer is found, it's often too late because the person wasn't able to afford a screening at the appropriate time. Screenings need to be made more accessible to those who may need them but aren't able to afford them. Additionally, people need to know how to recognize the signs that cancer may be developing within them. They need to be informed about how to feel for lumps or notice the changes in moles that may be dangerous. Help needs to be made more accessible.

Being accepted to participate in the ACTION (Appalachian Career Training in Oncology) Program has been what I would consider a blessing. I have always wanted to be able to help people. From a young age, I wanted to help better the lives of others. Since childhood, I've loved solving puzzles and problems. Cancer research is the perfect blend of both puzzles and problem-solving. My first choice would have never been cancer research; I have always wanted to be in the emergency room or in the operating room, helping patients hands-on. Although working in the ER does save lives and puts smiles on patients' faces, it doesn't measure up to the amount of joy that would come from helping to cure cancer. I've personally watched cancer pull my family apart piece by piece. I've seen my best friend's mother survive breast cancer. I've seen one of my high school friends face highly advanced testicular cancer, beat it, and still get accepted into Princeton University in just nine months. These things are the things that make me want to pursue a career in oncology and cancer research. Though other careers are just as rewarding, save just as many lives, and help just as many people, cancer research has a close place to my heart. I want to help change the outcome for those grandparents who want to watch their family grow, for the mothers and fathers who have children to guide through life, and for the brothers and sisters who have to be lifelong best friends to one another. Family and friends are what surround a person's heart, and cancer shouldn't be the thing that takes them away. The ACTION Program is supporting that dream to help people and prevent cancer from destroying more families, as it did mine.

Notes

1. Cancer Facts & Figures, 2019, retrieved July 10, 2019, from Cancer.org website, https://www.cancer.org/research/cancer-facts-statistics/all-cancer-facts-figures/cancer-facts-figures-2019.html.

2. "Stats of the States—Cancer Mortality," 2019, retrieved July 10, 2019, from https://www.cdc.gov/nchs/pressroom/sosmap/cancer_mortality/cancer.htm.

3. "Explore Smoking in Kentucky. 2018 Annual Report," 2018, retrieved July 10, 2019, from America's Health Rankings website, https://www.americashealthrankings.org/explore/annual/measure/Smoking/state/KY.

4. "Obesity and Cancer," 2011, retrieved July 10, 2019, from National Cancer Institute website, https://www.cancer.gov/about-cancer/causes-prevention/risk/obesity/obesity-fact-sheet#q4.

5. "Pneumoconiosis," 2015, retrieved July 10, 2019, from American Lung Association website, https://www.lung.org/lung-health-and-diseases/lung-disease-lookup/pneumoconiosis/.

Cancer Is Not a Vacation

Solomon Patton

HELLO, READERS. I bet you have already read a couple of my classmates' stories about how cancer has affected their lives in some way, or you are just reading mine because you know of me and are from Carter County. Or maybe it's because you live in Olive Hill, where we have only a McDonald's and Subway, and I can't forget the ole Mexican restaurant that sits on the corner. Well, first I would like to introduce myself; my name is Solomon Davis Patton. I have two amazing parents named Heath and Christy Patton, and I have three sisters named Hayla, Hadessah, and Aalyah Patton. Oh, wait, I can't forget my three dogs named Luna, Penelope, and Drew. Well, that's enough about me, how about I tell you why and how cancer has affected my life tremendously?

My great-grandmother died after having cancer for only a short time. I was only four when she passed away, and she spent many of her last days in her home while my grandmother cared for her. My grandmother was also later diagnosed as having precancerous breast tissue and opted to have a double mastectomy because two of her sisters had previously died from breast cancer and her other two sisters were diagnosed and treated. Well, there I was at the age of four, I was spending every day out at my great-grandmother's house with my best friend at the time, Cora Burton, and every time I asked my grandmother what was wrong with her, she said she had cancer. At the time, when I was four, I thought cancer was a vacation a lot of old people took, but I soon realized this was real serious when I hugged her for the last time at the hospital. Another side to the story is that this affects both sides of my family tremendously. My dad's side of the family has a long line of cancer, like stomach and skin cancer. Even though

I barely knew this side of the family, it still breaks my heart to hear about how they have suffered through this pain called cancer.

I think that cancer and other illnesses like this are starting to become more and more prevalent as time has gone on. Thirty years ago, we would have to go halfway across the country to find some twelve-year-old with cancer, but now I just have to look in the place I call home with a population of 1,600 people to find people with cancer. Many wonder why this is such a big issue, and I can answer that one really quick. It is because of our high school and middle school teachers. I think I can say this on behalf of all the student body of West Carter High School, where approximately 50 percent of students chew/smoke. One of the teachers on May 23, 2019, said, "Anyone need a can to spit in?" I think instead of worrying about our ACT scores, we should focus on our health. Did you know that chew has thirty chemicals in it that cause cancer? That is not counting the other thousand that don't cause cancer but still harm you in some way. Some parents are like, "No, this can't be my kid," but I hate to break it to you but it very well could be. Hey, local news channels, how about instead of showing us stuff that is useless to the human mind and pointless politics hating on our president, show us how the kids of and around Kentucky and the United States are smoking and chewing stuff that will ruin your gums, lungs, and bodies and might even kill you. How about showing how teachers are offering students cans to spit their spit into. On the smoking side of things, in the past year vaping, or better known as Juuling (this is a huge e-cigarette company), has taken Carter County schools by storm. Instead of playing in gym class, kids go to the locker rooms and Juul. If you are about the age of thirty you have probably heard of vaping on the news. But most of you have no idea what it is. The National Cancer Association says, "JUULing refers to using one brand of e-cigarette called JUUL, which is popular among kids, teenagers and young adults. JUULs are small, sleek, high tech-looking and easy to hide. They look like USB flash drives and can be charged in a computer. JUULs can be hidden in the palm of the hand and are hard to detect because they give off very little vapor or smell. Kids and teenagers are known to use them in school restrooms and even in the classroom." So now you know what Juuling is, but do you know what it does to your kids? There has been a debate about whether Juuling is less harmful than smoking regular cigarettes, but there have been many recent deaths and illnesses associated with such products and the long-term ef-

fects of e-cigarette products are not yet known.[1] This happened with cigarettes and chewing tobacco, whose long-term effects were not known when
they first came out. But I can promise you in the future that this will be a
big deal, just like when they found out chewing tobacco causes cancer after
it became popular with teens. This is when the tobacco companies were
forced to start printing "This product causes gum cancer" on the side of the
can. I predict in ten years Juuling will be the same.

I think this is a big deal, and organizations like the Centers for Disease
Control and Prevention have been trying to crack down on the drugstores
and gas stations for selling Juul pods (the part of the Juul that contains the
juice that has the flavor and the cancer-causing chemicals). I did a survey
at school, and all of the kids that I surveyed have vaped or own a Juul, and
75 percent of the twenty are all underage and have bought Juul pods from a
gas station. You might be thinking, "Wow, Carter County is really screwed
up," but from talking to my twenty classmates from the Markey Cancer
Center Appalachian Career Training in Oncology (ACTION) Program, I
know that this is happening all over the state. Chris Prichard and Dr. Nathan Vanderford told me to get the community involved to help address
these problems.

Do you know what is a really big problem in Carter County (besides
the lack of fast food restaurants and people)? It is breast cancer. I think
the reason this is such a big deal is because most people in Carter County
don't breastfeed their children. You might be thinking to yourself, "Wow,
Solomon, that statement was out there." Well, studies show that women
that have breastfed their kids are less likely to get or have breast cancer.
For example, my best friend's mom has gone through breast cancer. She
has two kids, and neither one was breastfed. The American Cancer Society
states that mothers who breastfeed lower their risk of pre- and post-meno-
pausal breast cancer. Most women who breastfeed experience hormonal
changes during their periods. This reduces a woman's lifetime exposure
to hormones like estrogen, which can promote breast cancer cell growth.[2]

My third point is that kids these days don't really know what cancer is.
A lot of people think they know what cancer is, but they don't know the actual definition. The actual definition is a disease caused by an uncontrolled
division of abnormal cells in a part of the body. Like most of you, I didn't
know what cancer was two months ago. When I was four, I thought cancer

was a vacation. Now that I know the real definition, I cannot wait to inform my school and my community about cancer and how to prevent it.

Cancer is something that I want to shine a light on in my county and all of the fifty-four Appalachian counties in Kentucky. I would be honored to come to your school and give a speech about how Juuling and teen tobacco use is ruining the great state of Kentucky—the place I and so many other great individuals call home.

Wow, what a trip this has been. I am on my last week here in the AC-TION summer program, and I have had my ups and downs from arguments with people over how to act around certain people and other petty things. But this has truly been amazing. I have learned so much from my mentors in my lab, and now they are like my friends. When I first came to the University of Kentucky, I had really narrow views about immigration, but after speaking with my lab mentors about their struggles with getting their U.S. citizenship after they have worked here and had kids here, I think that we should work on our immigration policies in the United States—but that is for another time.

I would like to thank Mr. Chris Prichard and Dr. Nathan Vanderford for this amazing opportunity to come on board and learn so much valuable information about cancer. I cannot wait to see where this path will take me.

Notes

1. American Cancer Society, *What Do We Know About E-Cigarettes?* 2019, retrieved from American Cancer Society, https://www.cancer.org/cancer/cancer-causes/tobacco-and-cancer/e-cigarettes.html.

2. American Cancer Society, *Lifestyle-related Breast Cancer Risk Factors*, 2019, retrieved from American Cancer Society, https://www.cancer.org/cancer/breast-cancer/risk-and-prevention/lifestyle-related-breast-cancer-risk-factors.html.

The Question

Brianna Reyes

I'VE COME TO find that questions are often more powerful than answers. To be more specific, it's through our questions that we find ourselves starting on trails and paths we could have never imagined if it hadn't been for our curiosity. One memorable question formed during my time in elementary school was, "Who do I want to be when I grow up?" That simplistic question has remained in the back of my mind, following me everywhere I turn. That question has walked with me through various birthdays and many nights of tossing and turning. It's an unavoidable question that nearly everyone will face at some point in their life. At first, our answers may consist of our dream occupations such as superhero, doctor, mother, and so on. Fortunately, our overall destiny always puts us in a position to save, take care of, and help others. It appears that we find our truest passions when increasing the quality of life for one another. From the time I was a little girl, all I could perceive myself being was someone who cared greatly for those around me. I've answered the question of who I want to be hundreds of times, in numerous ways with countless opportunities in mind. Who I am has always been knitted into the inspiration I've felt when hearing stories of people who help others. Part of me believes that everyone, at least at some point in their life, aspires to lift someone up and help them. Many people follow their childhood initiative to be a blessing to those around them, while others decide against it. However, as for me, Brianna Haleigh Reyes, my long-awaited answer to my childhood question has shown me what I'm searching for just may be found in a medical-related career.

My question has brought me through many different journeys. It's shown me that I value wholesome living and the wholehearted loving of people. It has brought to my attention that I can't be someone who will just "work a job" for the rest of my life; I wish to make an even greater impact. I want to be who I wish I had had in my life while I was growing up. My question brought me down a small street in Grayson, Kentucky, where I found a United Pentecostal Church. I was led to an amazing group of people who love and support me. They showed me that we don't live for ourselves; instead, we live to help those who are in need, and we strive to be a light to those who live in a constant state of darkness. I find contentment in knowing that I helped make a difference in another person's life. To pursue a career in which my entire life is devoted to making a difference would only make sense. I am uncertain about the specifics, but I know my niche will be found in the medical field. In addition to giving my question the power to direct me, applying my ability to learn, and using my heart, I feel that the area of cancer is beginning to beckon me.

Fortunately for my interest, in April 2019 I was accepted into the Appalachian Career Training in Oncology (ACTION) Program. This program has allowed me to get a firsthand experience with cancer research and many other careers in the oncology field. It has also allowed me to remain on the University of Kentucky campus for a total of five weeks. During these five weeks, I worked with the Total Cancer Care (TCC) team, also known as ORIEN, the Phase I Clinical Trial team, and so many more outstanding teams and individuals. I observed different surgeries and learned very helpful information throughout our scheduled workshops. Being part of this program has given me a great deal of respect for those who help take care of others and a great deal of respect for those who have been in battle with cancer. Experiencing something goes so much deeper than just having knowledge of something.

This being said, cancer is an extreme burden that has struck fear of the unknown into many; if it hasn't for you, it most certainly has for someone close to you. Ambrose Redmoon once stated, "Courage is not the absence of fear, but rather the judgment that something else is more important than fear." Many fight off their fear with courage and hope, but that doesn't mean this disease leaves them with peaceful thinking. Cancer doesn't just steal one's health; it steals their promised future, their aspirations, and sometimes even their faith. Although I have no direct experience with cancer in my immediate family, I can see the drastic amount of pain that cancer brings upon our society. From children who never make it to adulthood, to adults who never get to see their golden years, cancer is taking the lives of many, as it has been for some time now. I feel the urge to help when I look into the somber eyes of people around me who have lost a family member to a battle with cancer. Cancer doesn't just affect an individual; it affects a family, a home, and so much more. My experience is expressed through the sympathy I feel for those who have had crippling heartache due to this ungracious disease.

While living in Eastern Kentucky, I have been made aware of the destructive habits formed in this area. I see numerous people daily who are carrying around a pack of cigarettes or a can of chewing tobacco. Even in my high school, many kids I know are now using e-cigarettes or chewing tobacco long before the legal age, which doesn't make it any better. It's quite common to be exposed to different people who use tobacco frequently, seeing that it is ranked among the top ten cash crops in Kentucky according to norml.org.[1] Because Grayson, Kentucky, is a very agricultural and blue-collar type of city, I've come to find that I'm never too far from a field of tobacco. It seems as if everywhere I turn, everyone has learned to accept it because it's part of the cultural background. Thankfully, this hasn't gone unnoticed in my community. Throughout my schooling, I've been informed of risk factors that have the potential to cause cancer and the severity of the impact they cause. There are various awareness projects and programs that I've attended, even as early as fifth grade, about the harmful effects of tobacco, e-cigarettes, and drug abuse. Although the problem has been around for years, people are still working on new ways to address and inform people about the causes and effects of cancer.

As well as presentations done by many educated individuals, I believe social media has somewhat exposed me to this disease as well. Being interactive on Facebook will show you a vast number of people who are battling different types of cancer. I frequently stumble upon a fundraiser contributing to someone in need of help to afford their chemotherapy. People have sent me numerous invites to different events that are raising awareness of cancer. Media connects people in various ways. It is one venue that has exposed me to several manifestations of cancer—from friends asking for prayers for their loved ones to Facebook videos of people sitting by hospital beds singing along with their family members before they pass away. Media reveals the raw and real emotion formed from a cancer diagnosis. I believe exposure to something can and will cause a burden to form inside of you.

The more conversations and survivor testimonies I read or hear relating to cancer, the more of a tug I feel. Although my experience with cancer is not direct, I still feel a nudge to keep searching in order to do something more than what we've already done. Our society often believes, "If I'm not directly affected by this, it doesn't matter." That mentality shows a pure lack of sympathy and a large disregard for the value of one's well-being. Even if it's just one person who struggles, we should fight for them harder than cancer fights against them.

My old Kentucky home will always be home to my heart. It's housed many people throughout time. Having said this, in any loving home, it's important to take clear notice of what is in proper order and what needs a little maintenance. Cancer in Kentucky comes through many veins of life and comes in many conditions, some more violent than others. To take notice of cancer in Kentucky means that I see there are a lot of people who do it right by valuing and taking care of themselves, but still get an unexpected diagnosis. Noting this, I understand cancer doesn't discriminate; no matter your age, race, or income, there's always a chance of getting it somehow, someway. Cancer is something that can come unexpectedly and suddenly. It does not come for people only of a certain social status, religion, or anything else for that matter. I may not understand every in and out of why people get cancer yet, but I see its prevalence in the area around me.

Furthermore, there are hundreds of different contributors to the development of cancer. As previously stated, I don't live far from a tobacco field. Any direction I turn, chances are, there is a tobacco field from five to ten miles away. The tobacco fields are an observable channel through which cancer sneaks its way into our community. People mostly smoke and chew tobacco, despite the obvious cancer warning signs right on the label; smoking is the equivalent of running a red light or a stop sign, in my opinion. I believe that any lifestyle or habit that involves a consistent use or the involvement of something known to be cancer-causing is a major detriment in Kentucky. The main supervillain I see in the lives of those around me are tobacco products.

In addition to the use of tobacco, farmers usually don't seem to wear proper protective clothes to fight off ultraviolet (UV) radiation. Lots of tobacco farmers work long days in the harsh heat. If a farmer doesn't use sunscreen or proper protection from the UV rays, there's a higher risk that they will get skin cancer. Not only farmers, but construction workers are at a higher risk as well. Reflection of the sun off brighter surfaces, such as concrete or metal, can increase your overall sun exposure. From farmers to construction workers, the sun is yet another overall cause of cancer. Kentucky has more farms than I could count and has even more roadways that are continuously being worked on in the summertime. Anyone employed in outdoor work in the scorching sun is at risk if they aren't taking the proper precautions.

I never like pointing out issues if I can't take the time to consider a solution. As for the issues I've previously listed, there are already many options for a solution. Fortunately, from many years of research, people are forming ideas, creating programs, and taking the initiative to alleviate the issues we have at hand. To really address some forms of cancer in Kentucky, it takes looking at the toxicity of the routines by which hundreds live. People in Eastern Kentucky have always been raised around rough work outside. I believe a change in industry could occur if people with authority used their efforts to help farmers find a different cash crop to sell. To prevent skin cancer, I believe it should be considered as a state law for labor employers to keep plenty of sunscreen on hand for their employees. Along with this, the apparel of labor workers should be reconsidered to find light protective clothes that cover the entire body to limit prolonged exposure to the sun.

In summary, in my efforts to stress the broadness and the immense topic of cancer, I have merely listed a few causes as well as a few solutions while providing background about who I am. However, I am a person living in a world where cancer does, in fact, exist. It isn't beautiful, but the people affected are. I aim to involve myself in the fight against cancer in any way that I can. My heart is motivated by the sense of destiny created by the small, yet impactful question of my future purpose. My hope and prayer are that more questions are asked about this topic around the world and that more people find out that their curiosity leads them to a career in the cancer-related medical field.

Notes

1. NORML Foundation, *Kentucky Top 10 Cash Crops,* 1997, retrieved from NORML, https://norml.org/legal/item/kentucky-top-10-cash-crops.

What Cancer Is in My Life

Megan Schlosser

MY NAME IS Megan Ann Rose Schlosser, and I am from Somerset, Kentucky. I go to Southwestern High School, and I belong to the graduating class of 2022. When I graduate, I would like to pursue a career as either an obstetrician, a pediatrician, or an endocrinologist. An obstetrician is a doctor who concentrates on childbirth, pregnancy, and postpartum periods. A pediatrician is very similar to an obstetrician but works with children ages infant through twenty-one. Toward a different side of the medical world, I would also like to be an endocrinologist. Endocrinologists deal with hormones and the endocrine system no matter what a patient's age is. I would love to attend the University of Kentucky to fulfill these dreams. I would like to be an obstetrician or a pediatrician because I love taking care of children and seeing them happy. To be able to help bring a baby into the world would just be an amazing experience. I also have a really close relationship with my pediatrician, and I would love to be just like her. The reason I want to be an endocrinologist is that I have an endocrine disorder: a medical condition called diabetes insipidus (DI). This is a disorder in which you have increased salt and water metabolism followed by increased urination. I am hoping that this will give me a better personal understanding about endocrine problems and help me pursue my dream of becoming a doctor.

The reason why I would like to go into the medical field is that it really interests me and grabs my attention. I always thought about becoming a doctor ever since I was in seventh grade when I was selected to be a part of the medical honors class. In this class, we researched diseases and learned about the different tools doctors use on a daily basis. My favorite part, the part that really sparked my interest in the medical world, was at the end of the term when we got to dissect a sheep's brain. It was loads of fun, and I would definitely recommend it for anyone who may have an interest in the human body and how it works.

After attending the medical class in seventh grade, I continued my medical pathway once I reached high school. In high school, I took two medical classes: anatomy and bio-med. In anatomy, we learned about the body's structure. I was scared of being in this class because I was surrounded by upperclassmen, but it was one of my favorite classes I have taken in my entire life. I wouldn't say the class was easy, but I picked up fairly quick on the medical terminology, which in turn gave me an advantage in bio-med. Bio-med was different from anatomy. In bio-med, instead of learning about the structure, we learned more about the functions of the body and different diseases and disorders. The teacher in bio-med was also the person running the HOSA (Health Occupations Students of America) club. In this club we learned and studied what the medical field would be like. Toward the end of the year, we all packed up and went to a HOSA conference. The HOSA conference involved a lot of medical challenges, either hands on or on paper, in which students were allowed to participate. For those not competing in the HOSA conference, there were educational showings or opportunities to be part of the Courtesy Corp and help with student testing. Even though I didn't compete, I still learned a lot of valuable information about cancer and the medical field in general, and I will definitely try to compete next year.

Cancer is not new to me. The people that cancer has taken from me have been the people who have changed me the most as a person. My pediatrician, who developed breast cancer, took care of me since I was a baby. She taught me to never give up and to be kind. She was the kindest person anybody could ever know because she always had a smile on her face with a joke to follow. Her presence was always bright, even at work where she worked really hard for what she had. She fought the bitter battle against breast cancer to the very end and never gave up. She kept her hopes high and attitude positive about the situation better than anyone could have. Everyone loved her, and we all miss her being with us.

My aunt Crickett also battled bladder cancer. She beat it her first time around, but cancer sometimes finds a way back. It is relentless. She was always so bold and outgoing and did not care what anybody thought of her. She taught me to have fun as a kid, to live life to the fullest, and to not let anybody tell me what I can't do. She made going to family events ten times better, especially on the Fourth of July when she came to visit from Tennessee.

Additionally, another one of my beloved family members who will be remembered is my uncle Thurman. Uncle Thurman has a very special place in my heart. I was the very first newborn baby he ever held, so after that we were practically inseparable. He was your typical hillbilly. He was always shouting in his really strong country accent, riding around on his four-wheeler with his dog, Holly, on the back, and going to see his sister whom he loved and cherished. Even though he was a country bumpkin, he had a huge heart and believed in me. He always used to say, "EYE, MEG I AM PROUD OF YOU AND ALL THAT OTHER STUFF," then laugh it off. He has always been proud of me and what I was becoming in life. We always had a special bond, even up to the end.

In November 2017, we found out that he had cancer and that it had spread to his brain and his bones. The doctors said he had a couple months to live, but sadly, we had only a few weeks. He passed and went on to a much better place on January 11, 2019. Before he died, he worried about his dog, which he had taken care of and watched grow. He wanted someone who would love her and take care of her with ease. Now, Holly wasn't like any other dog; she was a very fat, prideful, and sassy Jack Russell and chihuahua mix. I felt that the person he wanted to take Holly in was me. So I took her in, and I have no regrets. I love her with all my heart, as he did. He has taught me to always take pride in what I do, just like Holly. Sadly, on June 30, 2019, at the age of fourteen, she went to a better place to reunite with my uncle Thurman.

Cancer is, in my opinion, the worst disease in the world. It affects not just the patients and the family but also their doctors, nurses, and friends. I would like to say thank you to all the doctors and nurses for their services and sacrifices they make for every patient. It takes a lot for a person to put someone else before themselves. We all, even the doctors and nurses, have at least one person that we wish we could say thank you to. I feel that usually the people that cancer takes are the ones who have an upbeat attitude and who have impacted everyone in a positive way.

In the United States of America, Kentucky is the most impacted by cancer out of all other states.[1] The most closely related reasons for the incidence of cancer are smoking, diabetes, and physical inactivity. The most prevalent type of cancer in Kentucky is lung cancer. Lung cancer is the most common because a large number of people smoke cigarettes and use other tobacco products.[2] About 32 percent of all cancers can be traced back to tobacco substances, and 80–90 percent of lung cancer is caused by smoking.[3] The sad thing about it is that deaths caused by smoking and using tobacco products are preventable. Diabetes can also cause you to develop cancer. According to WebMD, "Diabetes can cause pancreas, liver, and endometrial cancer to form, and it doubles the risk. Colorectal, breast, and bladder cancer can increase in probability by 20% to 50% because of diabetes. Diabetes in one aspect can be beneficial. It can cut the risk of men getting prostate cancer by nearly half."[4] "The top 5 deadliest cancers are lung, colon, breast, pancreatic, and prostate," according to LiveScience.[5] Prostate is a very common type of cancer for men. Its incidence rate is close to that of breast cancer in women.

Since tobacco is a cash crop in Kentucky, I believe it's going to be tough to have people stop smoking. Smoking is an example of an environmental factor that causes cancer. Another risk factor is living in a rural area. If you live in a rural area, mortality rates for lung, prostate, and colon cancer are higher than in urban areas. Another factor that can affect whether a person will get cancer is genetics. This is one of the few causes of cancer that is nonmodifiable. There are many DNA mutations in genes that can raise your risk for cancer. In Kentucky, we have so many risk factors that could cause this disease to form.

I believe if more people in Kentucky had a better education about cancer, then we could protect ourselves. Any amount of tobacco use is bad, even just a little. If people learn what these harmful factors are like tobacco, we might be able to help one another as a community.

Anyone can get cancer. Most people have the mindset of "not me," thinking that they will not be the one that will get some form of cancer. We need to realize that anyone can get it. Your friends, your neighbors, your family, or even you are at risk. So if we, as a community, could pull together and explain and warn everyone and anyone we know about cancer, we could save the people we love. To protect Kentucky's citizens and Kentucky's children, we need to come together and not be afraid to speak out against cancer-causing habits, ingredients, and exposures. The more we educate, the better off society will be.

Notes

1. Centers for Disease Control, https://www.cdc.gov/nchs/pressroom/sosmap/cancer_mortality/cancer.htm.

2. American Cancer Society, https://www.cancer.org/cancer/cancer-causes.html.

3. https://www.cdc.gov/tobacco/data_statistics/fact_sheets/health_effects/effects_cig_smoking/index.htm.

4. D. J. DeNoon, "Why Does Diabetes Raise Cancer Risk?" June 16, 2010, retrieved from https://www.webmd.com/diabetes/news/20100616/why-does-diabetes-increase-cancer-risk.

5. A. Chan, "The 10 Deadliest Cancers and Why There's No Cure," September 10, 2010, retrieved from https://www.livescience.com/11041-10-deadliest-cancers-cure.html.

It Can't Happen to Me

Kaitlin Schumaker

MOST OF MY friends call me by my last name, Schumaker, but my full name is Kaitlin Schumaker. I'm a sixteen-year-old student entering my junior year at North Laurel High School and the Center for Innovation. I live on a farm in East Bernstadt, Kentucky, the northern tip of Laurel County in the southeastern region of the state. Our county is named after the mountain laurel trees that grow here, and the county is well known for our annual Chicken Festival, since Kentucky Fried Chicken originated here.

The number twelve comes up a lot throughout my family. For example, my grandparents were married on December 12, 1996; I was born almost seven years later on February 12, 2003; and exactly twenty months later my sister was born on October 12, 2004. I have thought about many career paths since childhood, and thankfully, I have seen the errors in those career plans while I have found one that is more suited to my interests: forensic pathology. A TV show, *The Forensic Files*, actually introduced me to this profession, and I was quickly drawn to figuring out more about this potential career. I went from watching *The Forensic Files* in my spare time to checking out books about forensic pathology from the local library. This finally led me to the conclusion that I would like to spend the rest of my life doing something that revolves around that topic.

In addition to my family connection with the number twelve, there sadly seems to be another connection with cancer. A great portion of my family has been diagnosed with this disease: my mom had melanoma, my nana had ovarian cancer, and my great-grandma had breast cancer. We are very grateful that all of those cases had positive results and, in most instances, were caught early. For example, my great-grandma surprisingly found out that she had breast cancer after a car door hit her in the chest and left a bruise that wouldn't heal. After much convincing, she went to the doctor and was later diagnosed with breast cancer and was informed that the car door literally saved her life. If it hadn't hit her, the cancer would not have been detected as early. With less than a dozen chemotherapy sessions, her cancer went into remission.

Unfortunately, not all stories play out like that one. Seven days after submitting the paperwork to apply to this program, my grandpa Jones passed away from invasive liver cancer. Two weeks before his untimely passing, Grandpa Jones had walked into the Veterans Affairs Hospital in Lexington because he was experiencing breathing problems. At the time, this was not out of the ordinary because he had COPD (chronic obstructive pulmonary disease) and was trying to get oxygen approved for his home. What started out as just one of his monthly hospital visits became a more extended stay as they found a mass on his liver and did a biopsy.

After he healed from this procedure, he returned home and got a call from the hospital about his results two days later. He was informed that his cancer was already at a stage at which the treatments could only prolong his life for a few months at best, not cure it. With this in mind, he declined any treatments that the center offered. This, of course, did not help his condition, and his health declined rapidly. In a matter of a few days, he went from walking on his own to needing assistance to move around. Soon after, he was completely bed bound. In his last few days, there were many false alarms when his nurse thought that he was going to die, and everyone would rush over just to see that my grandpa was still holding on.

On the day of his death, I hoped that it was just another false alarm when we got the call from the nurse. But we had been there for five hours, and he was still breathing shallowly. My sister, Grace, and I had not left the room for the entire visit, so we walked out for a few minutes with my mom to get a breather. In this timespan, his breaths became even shallower, and by the time we reentered the room, my grandpa had just passed. All around me people were crying, wailing, murmuring Bible verses, in disbelief, but I also felt a closeness that I've never experienced before. His death brought my family together. In the following weeks after the funeral, all former arguments and disputes that had been going on for years were forgotten about and put on the side. It was the most peaceful I've ever seen my family. This peace didn't last forever, as life doesn't stop because of death. It's constantly moving regardless of what's occurring, but parts of the peace remained, and some of the tensions have been resolved. I know my Grandpa Jones would be happy that something good came out of this horrible situation.

"It can't happen to me." This five-word phrase could sum up half of Kentucky's cancer epidemic. While there are other factors that do contribute to this increasing problem, with more cases popping up each year, I feel that both a lack of information and misinformation really drive the cancer incidence. Most people in this region at least know someone who has suffered from cancer and have seen how it affected that person's family and their financial well-being. It's not that the citizens of these areas have no idea what cancer is or that certain factors, such as smoking, can increase your likelihood of being diagnosed. The issue is that many teenagers believe that they're on top of the world and that nothing bad can happen to them, which is obviously not true.

This is one of the reasons why this age group finds themselves in tough situations. This way of thinking doesn't go away as you get older and leave high school. People don't want to imagine something terrible could happen to them, so instead of taking preventive measures, they pretend that the possibility of being diagnosed with cancer is impossible.

This is a dangerous way to think as it puts people at higher risk, but it's not their fault. I think as human beings we try to distance ourselves from tragedies, as we don't know how to comprehend something like that happening to us. On the other hand, I feel that lack of information isn't as bad as the misinformation being shared. I've heard nonsensical theories on prevention such as taking showers once a month, to cancer being something that the government made up in order to scare people into getting vaccines. Once these conspiracy tales begin to circulate, they spread like wildfire. Most people in these regions take things like that with a grain of salt and don't believe them, but there are a select few who don't question any of it and end up spreading the misinformation around.

The overall environmental factors play a hand in the number of cancer cases here in Kentucky also. The Appalachian region is covered in coal mines that employ a portion of its citizens. These areas of employment are known to emit carcinogens that cause mutations in the lungs leading to such diseases as black lung and lung cancer. Additionally, in Eastern Kentucky, there are exposures that we experience from just walking outside, with air pollution, ultraviolet radiation, and asbestos. To make matters worse, there are not a lot of resources in these communities for the people to find ways around having to resort to methods that threaten them. For example, many people still burn tires instead of recycling them, thus putting more pollution into the air, or people refuse to have their homes checked for radon as they don't want to pay the fee.

These problems can be fixed with the right amount of outreach education, which would help reduce the gaps in information and would convey to the people of these areas that their actions have an impact on their health. This intervention would at the very least give them a general understanding of what's at stake and what they could do to decrease their chances of developing cancer. The purpose of this education would be to increase the overall awareness of the hazards that put you at risk for cancer and deplete the fake ones. Because younger people are more accepting to new ideas, the outreach initiatives would place a big focus on programs at schools. Children and teenagers would be able to form their own opinions about the topics being discussed. Hopefully, the programs would help educate them further on the matter, and in turn, they'll educate their parents. Even factors that we can't control, such as hereditary concerns, would be addressed to show how important it is to know your family medical history and how to take preventive measures.

Consequently, simple daily tasks can have lasting impacts. For example, not putting on sunscreen before spending time out in the sun puts you at risk for skin cancer. Active involvement with citizens can help change these behaviors and introduce the safer options that have little to no consequences. In addition to outreach, more availability of healthcare resources would encourage local residents to receive assistance and not be so wary of having simple procedures performed.

In these more rural areas, there are fewer hospitals, health education programs, and general healthcare. This healthcare disparity causes people to have to wait for extended amounts of time for treatment. Also, there's a lot of mistrust between the people and their doctors because while the doctors are telling their patients the truth, the patients see them as being cold and not on the same page for their needs. This mistrust between patients and healthcare providers causes patients to not seek out medical treatment unless it's absolutely necessary. By that time, the illness could have already progressed beyond the point of treatment. Even simple procedures like a colonoscopy or a prostate exam are met with great resistance as people don't want to be naked in front of medical staff or put to sleep with anesthesia. Lastly, there's also the fear of one of these procedures causing pain.

Of course, a patient's decision has to be respected, and we have to follow what they wish to happen. However, with the right amount of outreach information and with more accessibility to medical care, this decision has a higher chance of leading to a more successful outcome and a lower probability of becoming similar to what happened to my grandpa Jones. A general public that is educated is a reliable way to combat the cancer crisis, but there still need to be more localized forms of healthcare for a significant change to occur. Obviously, this change will not occur overnight, but with earnest involvement in these communities, this goal is possible for Kentucky to achieve.

Cancer
Kentucky's Disease

Spencer Shelton

EVERYONE KNOWS ABOUT cancer, and we need to stop it. My name is Spencer Ellis Shelton. I am from Whitley County, Kentucky, specifically from a small town called Williamsburg. I play soccer, tennis, and basketball. I have one sister, Rachel, who graduated on June 2, 2019, from Whitley County High School. Next school year, I will be a sophomore attending the same school, and I hope to graduate with high honors in the class of 2022. After high school, I want to be a doctor of any specialty, but I am especially interested in pediatrics. As with many others with this interest, children are of high value to me because they play the biggest role in our future. As long as I can help people become healthier, I will have purpose in such a workplace.

Kentucky has the highest cancer incidence and mortality rates in the country.[1] The way that cancer as a whole takes over Kentucky, specifically the Eastern or Appalachian area, is terrifying. Families are doused in losses, nearly each one with one or two people with a type of cancer that they know will either get the best of them or at least present itself as an obstacle for their work, their children, their hobbies, or their school. Patients see prayers go unanswered, and everyone watches them go downhill, unable to help. Cancer can put lives on hold. It is almost like pressing the pause button, forcing the patient to sit there, trying to move forward with life, just wanting to be past it all. Only some lucky people can resume, but there is permanent damage done. A person is changed forever.

An outline of what each ACTION (Appalachian Career Training in Oncology) Program participant was supposed to write for this essay said to include our personal experiences with cancer. I have too many to count.

They become forgotten sorrows for people who aren't too close to you, and you are lucky if there are people you *can* forget about, rather than those all too close. One personal example of a person close to me who had cancer is my grandfather. Around 2008, I was about six years old when my grandfather, J. T. Shelton, was diagnosed with early-stage prostate cancer. Cells from a kidney infection were tested, and they were deemed cancerous. After many consultations he decided to have his cancer removed, and later his entire prostate. He has since had cells taken from his head and arms to test, which have thankfully come back negative. Sometimes I think back to the screening and when he was diagnosed. Nothing else in his life seemed to matter then. Choices he made, the life he lived, the family he raised, or how many friends he had. Cancer didn't care.

The United States is certainly plagued by cancer. According to the National Cancer Institute (NCI), cancer incidence in the United States is 439.2 per 100,000 per year (based on 2011–2015 cases).[2] However, as stated above, cancer harms Kentucky more than any other state. It is the greatest emotional and, according to the CDC (Centers for Disease Control and Prevention), statistical bane of Kentucky's way of life.[3] Cancer is responsible for too many deaths, lives ruined or forever changed, and dreams given up on.

A few factors that increase the cancer rates in our state are tobacco use and lack of preventive screening. One type of tobacco use in Kentucky is smoking. Smoking is one of the most fundamental reasons why cancer reaches so many Kentuckians, especially on a rural level. For a long time, smoking has been a staple of Kentucky life. People have been smoking, becoming addicted to nicotine, and continuing to smoke for years. Not only that, but they are doing it around children and letting these children grow to become smokers. This vicious cycle—dare I call it a culture—continues to repeat itself over and over. Smoking has a direct correlation with lung cancer, unsurprisingly, which may be why it affects Kentucky at a rate higher than anywhere else in the United States.

Smokeless and chewing tobacco also stand out in Kentucky. Just because there is no smoke does not mean there is no risk. I can personally say that people start this habit very early, as students who attend my school regularly receive punishment for possessing or using chewing tobacco. Some of my friends from other schools even less fortunate than mine say they have seen their teachers using tobacco at school, which is obviously unacceptable. The tobacco industry will not give up on Kentucky, and we just can't seem to give up on tobacco.

Lack of screening for cancer also keeps many from knowing they have such a terrible ailment in the first place. Many types of cancer can be identified, and certain procedures similar to screenings can find changes the body makes prior to cancer formation, like polyps. Specifically, female cancer screenings like breast mammograms and pap smears are incredibly effective. However, with growing evidence that not enough people are receiving screenings, cancer continues to have its way with our state. This is why Kentucky is still maintaining a top spot in the numbers of cases of these two cancers.

Age might also contribute to this statistic. According to the NCI, one quarter of new cancer diagnoses are in people aged sixty-five to seventy-four.[4] I feel that many times, our older generation may feel that a vast number of symptoms are insignificant, causing them to ignore them. Most of the elders here simply grew up in a much tougher time and still feel that unless they are in dire conditions or are kept from working, they should tough it out and continue on with life. This often leads to stubbornness regarding recommended checkups and screenings. This lack of knowledge can delay medical and professional help until it is much too late. There is also the misconception factor about screenings, with people thinking that they may be very expensive or harmful. In reality, screenings are fairly affordable and very safe, and it could be argued that the result would be worth it regardless.

Thinking about how cancer continues to damage Kentucky, one might ask how we should combat it. What can we do to address cancer? For starters, if we cut tobacco use even just a little, the effects would be felt indefinitely. As I covered previously, smoking cigarettes and using smokeless tobacco both have been found to cause a varying list of cancers. In Kentucky, it seems to me that the amount of tobacco use is directly proportional to the growth of cancer rates. So naturally, it is evident that if we were to take a step back from tobacco as a state, it would be a massive step toward addressing cancer in Kentucky. I believe that this could also help many other places across the nation. Another way to help address cancer in Kentucky is to spread awareness and availability of cancer screenings. If rumors and misconceptions about cancer screenings were cleared up and people were taught that they may need screenings even though they don't feel any symptoms, a vast number of cases could be discovered, treated, and stopped before they could cause any harm. It is very important for our older generation to receive preventative screenings, as many types of cancer have recommended screenings annually once a patient is forty years of age or older. This is another problem that could be solved generally rather than just in the state of Kentucky.

To conclude, cancer in Kentucky is an immense problem. Lives are torn apart, and rifts are created in families, as with my family friend Jared, people I've never met, and even others I've forgotten. These personal stories show that cancer doesn't care about who you are or what you've achieved; it cares only about whether or not you can beat it. As the tobacco usage in our state and the lack of screenings continue, nothing will improve. However, if we spread positive awareness about the positives of screenings and promote them all while reducing tobacco use, the numbers could turn in our favor by a dramatic margin. If you see someone using tobacco, kindly tell them about the dangerous effects. You can also consider recommending screenings to friends and even get them yourself. Be the tool used to defeat cancer—for me, for you, for Kentucky.

Notes

1. C. Blackburn, "Cancer kills Kentuckians at highest rate (Update)," December 28, 2016, retrieved from https://www.naaccr.org/cancer-kills-kentuckians-at-highest-rate/.

2. Cancer Statistics, April 27, 2018, retrieved July 10, 2019, from https://www.cancer.gov/about-cancer/understanding/statistics.

3. L. Ramsey, "The CDC Just Mapped Which States Have the Highest Rates of Cancer in the US," May 8, 2017, retrieved from https://www.sciencealert.com/the-cdc-mapped-out-who-has-the-highest-rates-of-cancer-in-the-us.

4. Dana-Farber Cancer Institute, "Why Does Cancer Risk Increase As We Get Older?" May 18, 2017, retrieved July 9, 2019, from https://blog.dana-farber.org/insight/2016/06/why-does-cancer-risk-increase-as-we-get-older/.

You Never Plan for Cancer

Haleigh Thompson

FROM THE MOMENT you are a child and throughout your entire life, you have a designed plan for your future. This plan typically encounters alterations as you grow older and expose yourself to more of life. However, sometimes life exposes itself to you. These are the moments when your plan is forced to change. Nobody ever really anticipates these disturbances when arranging their future. Life throws them at you with no warning. They change everything.

My name is Haleigh Thompson, and my plan is to become a doctor. I am from Louisa, Kentucky, and I attend Lawrence County High School. My biggest aspiration for myself in life is to enter a medical-based career. For as long as I can remember, science has had a huge piece of my heart. Science never fails to amaze me, and I have such a deep passion to pursue it. The complexity of the anatomy and physiology of the human body intrigues me. I expect nothing short of being a successful doctor in the future. I have the drive and determination to achieve my goals and have taken the necessary steps toward doing so. I have shadowed a general surgeon, which solidified my desire for a future in medicine. I am currently a participant in the Markey Cancer Center's Appalachian Career Training in Oncology (ACTION) Program at the University of Kentucky. This program focuses on enhancing the knowledge of cancer among both participants and their communities. I am particularly interested in oncology for several reasons including my personal experience with cancer and my desire to combat the cancer epidemic of my home state, Kentucky.

Cancer is a very serious issue, especially in Kentucky. The state has the highest rate of cancer diagnoses as well as cancer mortalities. Lung, breast, and colorectal cancer are among the highest diagnosed.[1] Lung cancer is most closely related to smoking. A large number of individuals in Kentucky smoke tobacco, thus increasing the rate of lung cancer in the state. Smoking directly damages the lungs when inhaled. The more frequently one smokes, the more damage that occurs to the lungs. Cancer is developed when cells divide irregularly, forming a collection of cells referred to as a tumor. Smoking causes the cells that line the lungs to be damaged. Over time, the body becomes less able to repair the damaged cells. The chemicals found in cigarettes contain several cancer-causing agents. Additionally, secondhand smoke is a major issue. While someone may not personally choose to smoke, being exposed to others who do smoke can be dangerous as well because they are still inhaling a portion of the cancer-causing agents found in tobacco products.

Additionally, obesity is a major cancer-causing factor. Kentucky ranks eighth among states with the highest obesity problems.[2] The poverty seen in the area plays a large role in obesity rates. Eastern Kentucky is a socio-economically disadvantaged area. Because of this, more people eat inexpensive foods, such as junk food and fast food. This leads to obesity and potentially the development of cancer. The risk of breast, colorectal, and several other cancers present in Kentucky increases with obesity.[3] This is due to a variety of reasons, including increased levels of cancer-promoting factors.

Furthermore, I strongly believe that many residents of Kentucky lack general knowledge about cancer and cancer-causing agents. For example, many people in my personal life had no idea that Kentucky, their home state, has the highest rates of cancer in the United States. It is not unlikely that this also applies to many other people of Kentucky. Cancer is much too serious, and there is much too little awareness. To help remedy the problem of cancer in Kentucky, I believe awareness needs to be raised. The more people who are knowledgeable about the intensity and commonality of cancer, the more people who will make efforts to combat it. Awareness can be brought to the public through several different strategies. These include hosting events, distributing items such as key chains, and hosting cancer-awareness assemblies in schools. Youth are the future; it is very crucial that they are conscious of the issues surrounding cancer. I believe people of all ages need to gain insight about cancer, but the upcoming generations particularly do. With the youth being educated about cancer and how to help prevent it, there is a greater chance of cancer rates decreasing in the future.

I have witnessed the devastating effects of cancer firsthand. One of the most supporting, influential individuals present in my life is my sister, Amanda. She is thirty-three years old, from the small town of Fort Gay, West Virginia. Amanda and I are technically half-sisters with a seventeen-year age difference between the two of us. Despite this, we have an inseparable bond, one I would not trade for anything in this world. Almost all of my favorite memories include her. She is a genuine, caring woman who embodies one of the purest souls of anyone I know. Amanda has supported me in every aspect of my life, regardless of the circumstances. I wholeheartedly believe that there is not a single person who will have my back quite how she does. She has been, and continues to be, my biggest supporter in life. I consider myself very fortunate to have her as both my sister and my best friend. Everyone deserves an "Amanda" in their life.

Tuesday, January 24, 2017, was the most painful day of my life. I was wearing a brown sweater I had received as a Christmas present paired with my favorite shoes at the time. It's ironic how the days you want to forget the most are the ones you remember down to every last explicit detail. Although it was the peak of winter, my school was in session on this day. I arrived home from school in a mediocre mood. My day had been nothing fantastic, yet nothing terrible, or at least not yet anyway. I was completing homework for my reading class when my sister walked through the back door. Tears soaked her face, mascara running down her cheeks. My heart immediately fell to my feet. I knew something was horribly wrong. She finally managed to utter a sentence I wish I had never heard: "I have cancer." My sister had been diagnosed with stage 1 ovarian cancer.

A thousand worrisome questions crossed my mind: How serious is this? Can this be cured? Is this hereditary? What will happen in the future? How could something so terrible occur to someone so wonderful? I felt hopeless, unable to accept what I had just heard. In that moment, time had completely stopped. Not a word was spoken for at least five minutes. I think all of us had no idea how to react. Cancer does not give a warning of its arrival. There was no subtle entrance, no form of preparation. Cancer comes abruptly, often in the midst of pure bliss. What had begun as such a typical day transformed into a day filled with nothing but sorrow. My mind could not process what I had heard. If I was feeling all of these gut-wrenching emotions, I didn't even want to think of how she must have been feeling. I find it peculiar how several people can be in the same experience, yet all be impacted differently with a range of feelings. I remained strong for her sake. Amanda is such a support system for me; I had to be the same for her, regardless of how difficult this was. I had no idea of what the future held. My fears had overwhelmed me; I began to assume the worst of possibilities. One of the most difficult things I have ever done was hold onto hope in a period so far from hopeful.

Within stage 1 ovarian cancer, the cancerous cells are found present in the ovaries alone. This meant that the cancer had not yet metastasized to any other part of the body. This information was a slight silver lining. While the cancer was serious, it had not progressed to a completely despairing state. A course of treatment had to be chosen, and it had to be chosen quickly. If action was not taken soon, the cancer would spread, reaching a more critical stage. The smartest and most promising treatment was a hysterectomy. This is a surgical procedure in which the uterus and surrounding organs are removed from the body. With this, the possibility of childbirth is also removed.

At a ripe young age of thirty-one, my sister underwent a complete hysterectomy. This is so early in life to be faced with the consequences of the procedure. Typically, a complete hysterectomy would not be performed due to how young she was, but Amanda also had stage 3 endometriosis, a disorder affecting the uterus. Enduring both stage 1 ovarian cancer as well as stage 3 endometriosis, she had no other choice than a complete hysterectomy. She has no children and now has lost the ability to have any of her own. At the age of twenty-four, Amanda tragically experienced a miscarriage. I was seven at this time; therefore, I have little memory of how this affected her. However, I do know that deep down she secretly longed for a second chance at having children. This was taken away from her, and cancer is to blame. Witnessing the pain my sister experienced, both physically and emotionally, sparked a desire in me to pursue a career in healthcare.

On October 23, 2017, the hysterectomy procedure was performed. She was a high-risk patient for the surgery, but it was successful with no complications. This day was the exact definition of bittersweet. It was the day her cancer had been removed, but it was also the day she forever lost the ability to give birth. Throughout this melancholy time, my sister claimed not to be upset as one would assume. I saw past this; I knew she was breaking on the inside. I noticed the way in which she gazed upon happy families with children. Almost two years have passed since the surgery, and I still catch her doing so from time to time today. Children had always been sort of a taboo topic of discussion following the miscarriage. Any time someone brought children into discussion, she claimed that it wasn't very high of a priority for her. Although she hides it within her words, her actions reveal a hidden truth: she yearns to birth a child. My sister is the type of person who has so much compassion and empathy for others, but she bottles her own feelings inside herself. She supports anyone in her life, without expecting anything in return. I find it difficult to understand how she remains so strong throughout all the obstacles she has encountered. In such an emotionally deteriorating period of her life, my sister continued to be one of the strongest individuals I know. I admire the strength she encapsulates and hope to become even half as resilient of a woman as Amanda.

You plan your entire life: college, marriage, career, children.
Every goal and aspiration, perfectly aligned in a secured plan.
You plan your entire life, but you never plan for cancer.
Cancer changes every aspect of your arranged agenda in life,
causing you to question everything you once knew
Everyone hears the terrible stories of cancer and its diminishing effects.
But until it occurs in the midst of your own life,
it remains just that: a terrible story.
The harsh reality doesn't register in the human mind until experienced firsthand. Cancer delays any future plans.
Everything from that point onward in life revolves around cancer.
Even if the cancer is able to be treated, the fear of its return persists.
Life is never able to return to how it was,
how it was before cancer turned life a full 360 degrees.
Suddenly, you find yourself composing a new plan for yourself,
starting completely from square one.
You plan your entire life, but you never plan for cancer.

Notes

1. American Cancer Society, "Kentucky 2019 Estimates," accessed June 27, 2019, retrieved from https://cancerstatisticscenter.cancer.org/#!/state/Kentucky.

2. S. Kuhl, "Kentucky Ranked 8th-worst for Obesity," 2018, accessed June 27, 2019, retrieved from https://www.richmondregister.com/news/kentucky-ranked-th-worst-for-obesity/article_ab5b96c7-8978-5e36-9b7b-5a2c0905db13.html.

3. ASCO, "Obesity, Weight, and Cancer Risk," 2019, accessed June 27, 2019, retrieved from https://www.cancer.net/navigating-cancer-care/prevention-and-healthy-living/obesity-weight-and-cancer-risk.

Day In and Day Out

Ethan Tiller

ROBERT COLLIER SAID, "Success is the sum of small efforts, repeated day in and day out." My name is Ethan Tiller, and I will be a junior at East Carter High School during the 2019–2020 school year. I was born in Charleston, West Virginia, and moved to Grayson, Kentucky, at the age of two. I am sixteen years old and play varsity baseball and soccer. I play travel baseball in the summer for the Morehead War Eagles. All through school, I have maintained a 4.0 unweighted GPA, and I am currently tied for first place in the 2021 class. I enjoy being outside, and as a result, many of my hobbies are outside activities. Riding dirt bikes, four-wheeling, kayaking, fishing, boating, and many more things consume most of my free time. Additionally, I am involved in several clubs at school including Beta Club, Future Business Leaders of America, French Honors Society, Unite Club, and Unified Club. I am an ambassador for the Kentucky Special Olympics, and I travel around the state to teach other schools how to become a Unified Champion School. Unified Club promotes the inclusion of people with physical and/or mental disabilities.

Last summer, I was a teen volunteer at Cabell Huntington Hospital, where I worked in the Heart Catheterization Lab and the Sports Medicine Center. I was a recipient of the President's Volunteer Gold Service Award in 2018 for my volunteer activities such as feeding the homeless, building beds for the needy, participating in teen court, helping with the Special Olympics, and other efforts. Trying new things even when they seem challenging and unfamiliar is something I strive to do daily. A constant phrase I try to remember is "The only real mistake is the one from which we learn nothing," stated by Henry Ford.[1] Through my experiences, I've learned that when we embrace our differences, we grow as individuals and can celebrate achievements together.

I was born with a vascular malformation and have been under the care of doctors since birth. I have always felt such a deep appreciation of how much my healthcare providers cared about my desire to be an athlete and a "normal" kid. They have always made me feel that my childhood is just as important to them as it is to me. They have allowed me to be a part of the decision-making process with my care and potential treatment plans. From my perspective, these doctors and nurses are like superheroes who have the knowledge, power, and resources to fix any problem or to save anyone. My healthcare providers have impacted my life so much that I want to be able to make that same type of impact on the lives of others who may be facing similar challenges. Healthcare and medical professionals have always captivated my interest. The ability of professionals to quickly analyze and assess medical, ethical, and legal situations at just a moment's notice drives my interest even more. I love science, math, and engineering and have always enjoyed making a difference in people's lives, whether that be through volunteering, mentoring, or even through kindness. My goal is to be a doctor who will impact many different lives. I am undecided about which field of medicine; however, I hope my involvement in the Appalachian Career Training in Oncology (ACTION) and Rural Health Scholar programs will allow me to explore different career options.

In a small town, cancer affects not only family and friends but the entire community. This was amplified for my small town in Carter County when cancer struck the pastor of our church and high school team chaplain. Brother Paul Schmidt had an impact on everyone he met. His diagnosis of colon cancer took many people by surprise, including his own family. Even while fighting cancer, he seemed unaffected to the public. While Brother Paul was going through cancer treatment, he would FaceTime us during church services and talk about how he was doing with the treatment and anything he had been doing between the treatments. He was still able to make us laugh while he was fighting a physical and emotional battle with cancer. Even though he was in the hospital, Brother Paul still helped spread the gospel by praying and witnessing to other patients. These were just some of the many testaments he showed the church and community during this time. After a long battle, the Lord called him home. Cancer took someone close to everyone's heart in the area, and for me, it was the first time I lost someone so close. This experience opened many people's eyes to how horrible cancer is and how it can affect anyone.

Carter County seems to have an abundance of people who have been diagnosed with cancer in the last few years. Three of those people were my mother's friends, all of whom were younger than she, with young kids. Two of her friends were diagnosed with breast cancer, and one had ovarian cancer. One of them lost her battle last year to metastatic breast cancer that spread to her brain. There is a toddler from our area, diagnosed as a baby with pediatric brain cancer. Our entire town follows his health through Facebook and holds fundraisers to help his family during this time. I have a friend whose brother was diagnosed with brain cancer, and a teacher in our area lost her son to the same disease. My former basketball coach was recently diagnosed with aggressive brain cancer, and a school board member and father of one of my friends has brain cancer. Those numbers and the number of people whom I know that have battled cancer shock me. It is also shocking that cancer can happen to anyone regardless of their age, race, or gender. This led me to apply to the ACTION Program, so that I can gain knowledge about cancer prevention and hopefully raise awareness among people in my community.

My family is originally from the Appalachian area, with roots in Martin County and across the river in West Virginia. My great-grandma and great-grandpa, my great-uncle, my great-aunt, and many others all lost their battles with cancer. The majority of the cancer was tobacco-induced lung cancer, but others include breast cancer and prostate cancer. When my ancestors started using tobacco, they weren't aware that it would cause cancer. They ultimately paid the consequences of putting foreign substances into their lungs and their bodies. The other types of cancer could have been caused by their career or their location. Many of my ancestors were coal miners or lived in coal towns. Coal trucks passing their neighborhoods, schools, and creeks unintentionally released coal dust into the air, and coal contaminated the water where these people lived. There are also limited recycling centers in the Appalachian region, and people tend to pollute the air with harmful chemicals, such as oil or old cars or appliances in the creeks and rivers. It is also common practice to burn anything, such as tires, shingles, and old building materials, which could contain asbestos or lead paint.

Cancer is one of the scariest and most destructive diseases the body can have. Kentucky has the most cancer deaths in the country.[2] In 2019, there were ten thousand people in Kentucky alone who died from cancer. This leads me to believe that the main factor must be environmental. According to the Centers for Disease Control and Prevention (CDC), West Virginia and Kentucky have the highest rates of tobacco use in the United States.[3] One thing that the southern United States takes pride in is heritage, but taking pride in the heritage of tobacco use should not continue. Scientists and doctors alike have proved it causes cancer, yet people continue to use this harmful product. According to the American Cancer Society, Kentucky has the second-highest number of smokers in high school and over the age of eighteen, while also having a lower tax rate on tobacco than the national average. This creates a deadly combination, making the trend cheaper and easier to join.

Some people are different; they don't like the idea of tobacco. However, the companies make it harder and harder for them to resist nicotine. Vaping has swept the nation by storm, with people saying that vaping is not as bad as smoking tobacco. Vaping and Juuling have become extremely popular with young teens who never smoked cigarettes or used smokeless tobacco. It was originally marketed as "safe" and seemed like a cool thing to do. Because of the fruity and exotic flavors, it is not supposed to taste like tobacco. With limited research, it is hard to say what the effects of these products are or will be. Some studies have hypothesized that an effect of prolonged use could be "popcorn lung," which causes shortness of breath, damages small airways in the lungs, and results in coughing. Europe has already banned the use of some e-cigarettes or vapes because of the use of chemicals that have been proven to cause "popcorn lung," or bronchiolitis obliterans. San Francisco, the home of Juul Labs, became the first city in the United States to ban the use of e-cigarettes.[4] Many of the people who vape are unaware how much nicotine is truly in these e-cigarettes. Without this knowledge, people continue to use these products, becoming more and more addicted. Social media and the Internet could be in part to blame. Many public figures use tobacco or e-cigarettes, influencing younger generations. Young minds are malleable, creating habits and addictions that will be hard to break later. Our ancestors were in a similar situation when tobacco was introduced, and our generation will see the effects of vaping firsthand unless we can combat this epidemic.

Anyone who is from Kentucky knows that coal mining was a big part of our industry. Studies now show that inhalation of harmful chemicals released at some mines has resulted in mesothelioma: "the process of handling, grinding, cutting and crushing coal yields asbestos particles and coal dust particles. This puts coal miners at just as high of a risk for asbestos dust exposure as they have for coal dust."[5] The main cause of mesothelioma is asbestos or the inhalation of the substance. Asbestos is a known carcinogen in drywall, plastics, paints, and many more common items. The EPA actually allows for 1 percent use of asbestos in common items.[6] Most people probably don't know that these cancer-causing agents are in household items. The ACTION Program needs to spread awareness about this issue through our outreach portion of the program to educate people about these carcinogens.

Another contributing factor to the high cancer rates in Kentucky is obesity. Kentucky has the eighth-highest obesity rate in the country.[7] Kentucky also has the eleventh most fast food restaurants, at 4.8 per capita.[8] Also, the increase in fast food restaurants has resulted in the number of obese children tripling and the number of obese adults to rise by 17 percent.[9] Obesity has been known to increase cancer risk by up to 50 percent.[10] Part of the reason that fast food is so popular is that it is fast, tasty, and cheap. Because of supply and demand, farmers are forced to charge higher prices for naturally grown, non-GMO food. This makes fast food even more enticing. With Kentucky ranked the forty-fifth state in terms of median income, eating healthy just isn't feasible for some people and/or families.[11] Not only does high-priced natural food deter consumers, but it deters companies that might buy healthier food rather than processed food. This forces companies to use food that has been genetically modified, treated with pesticides, and made with anything else the producer decides to add to the product. Just as with vaping, putting foreign chemicals into our body can cause many problems. These chemicals could go as far as to change the sequences of DNA in our bodies, and if they don't, they can cause epigenetic modifications. Epigenetic modifications result when the DNA sequences remain unchanged but the gene function changes.[12]

Trends can have many different effects. Trends in tobacco use have caused many problems, but the ACTION Program could start a trend by helping get the community more involved and educated. Teens follow their peers like sheep follow a shepherd. This program is full of shepherds from all over Kentucky. I was one of the founding members of the Unified Club at our school. At first, it was hard and was met with some opposition. Two years later, students who use offensive language toward or about students with disabilities at our school are met with public shaming. The process of initiating the club took over two years and was all started by a few people who wanted something—unification between students—then reached out and obtained it. The ACTION Program is no different. With each member, we can bring back knowledge from the summer and share it with our schools, educate our communities, and make a difference one family at a time.

Since the beginning of this program, people have complimented and congratulated us. The community is excited that students in the area are doing something important like cancer research. Word spreads like wildfire, and parents start encouraging their children to get involved with similar programs. Students at every school are competitive, and when one student is involved in a program like ACTION, it motivates other students to make a difference. No student wants to be outdone by their peers, creating friendly competition. Not only will this benefit the students, but it will help the population as a whole better understand cancer.

Public outreach, a better understanding of cancer, and community involvement will help decrease cancer incidence and mortality in the great state of Kentucky. All of these aspects share a common thing: strength in numbers. The more people we can get involved in our goal of decreasing cancer incidence and mortality in Kentucky, the faster we can achieve that goal. The more people we can get into the labs, the more experiments we can perform. The more people fighting for change when it comes to tobacco use, fast food consumption, and harmful chemical pollution, the faster we can decrease cancer rates in Kentucky. With these small efforts, we will succeed and defeat cancer together.

Notes

1. Henry Ford, n.d., retrieved from https://www.goodreads.com/author/quotes/203714. Henry_Ford.

2. America's Health Rankings, 2019, retrieved from https://www.americashealthrankings.org/explore/annual/measure/CancerDeaths/state/KY.

3. Centers for Disease Control and Prevention, 2018, retrieved from https://www.cdc.gov/statesystem/cigaretteuseadult.html.

4. BBC, 2019, retrieved from https://www.bbc.com/news/business-48752929.

5. Mesothelioma Veterans Center, 2019, retrieved from https://www.mesothelio-maveterans.org/mesothelioma/causes/asbestos-exposure/occupations/miners/.

6. Mesothelioma + Asbestos Awareness Center (MAAC), 2019, retrieved from https://www.mesotheliomadiagnosis.com/asbestos/products/.

7. The State of Obesity, 2019, retrieved from https://www.stateofobesity.org/states/ky/.

8. Thrillest, 2018, retrieved from https://www.thrillist.com/news/nation/states-with-most-fast-food-restaurants-datafiniti.

9. National Collaborative on Childhood Obesity Research (NCCOR), n.d., retrieved from https://www.nccor.org/downloads/ChildhoodObesity_020509.pdf.

10. National Cancer Institute, 2017, retrieved from https://www.cancer.gov/about-cancer/causes-prevention/risk/obesity/obesity-fact-sheet.

11. Wikipedia, 2019, retrieved from https://en.wikipedia.org/wiki/List_of_U.S._states_and_territories_by_income.

12. Genetics Home Reference, 2019, retrieved from https://ghr.nlm.nih.gov/primer/howgeneswork/epigenome.

UNDERGRADUATE STUDENT ESSAYS

Appalachian Rose
Wilted by Geography

Lauren K. Collett

> Something is mine to do back in my own land. I don't know what yet, but I dream dreams . . .
>
> Mary C. Breckinridge

> The beginning lies in France perhaps. It must or I should not be here. But after that I know that the way leads back over the ocean to the country where my own children were born and where they are buried.
>
> Mary C. Breckinridge

I WAS BORN on October 17, 1997, at the Mary Breckinridge Hospital in the mountains of Appalachia in Hyden, Kentucky. I attended Hyden Elementary, Leslie County Middle School, and Leslie County High School. I played basketball, softball, and volleyball, and I was the valedictorian of my senior class. I am now a third-year, pre-medicine, biology major at the University of Kentucky, as well as a Robinson Scholar. I am also a member of the University of Kentucky Markey Cancer Center Appalachian Career Training in Oncology Program in which I participate in cancer-related observation, outreach, and research. In my free time, I enjoy volunteering with Kids Cancer Alliance at Indian Summer Camp and Bluegrass Care Navigators Hospice in Hyden and Hazard. I also enjoy traveling, whether it be to Ecuador for a health brigade or to New Orleans for the 14th Annual New Orleans Summer Cancer Meeting. I have a passion for learning about Appalachian cancer disparities, and my goal is to attend medical school to become an oncologist and to return home to serve Appalachia.

Growing up, I stayed with my mamaw and papaw, Irene and Odell Brock, while my mom worked. Mamaw had short, voluminous brown hair that always lay perfectly around her glass-framed, icy blue eyes and full, blushed cheeks. Her voice was smooth and calming like the complete silence that caresses your ears in the peace of your bedroom after hours of ear-wrenching noise. She was soft-spoken and mild-mannered, and her laugh was like the soft giggle of a small schoolgirl up to no good. Papaw had dark skin and hair like his Native American ancestors who came before him, accompanied by stunning blue eyes and a smile that was contagious. He loved to dance, sing, and play while Mamaw shook her head and occasionally cracked a smile.

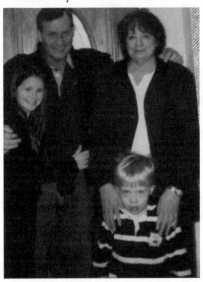

At a young age, Papaw taught me to whistle like the birds, catch tadpoles in the creek, and change gears on a stick shift, while Mamaw taught me to read words from a random list she made on her 8″ x 3″ notepad, to write in cursive, and to play the piano—all before I started preschool. In addition to all the teaching and learning, every day, Mamaw and I walked hand in hand through the yard with a watering pot, sprinkling lukewarm well water over the colorful petals of our favorite flowers. Life was great at Mamaw and Papaw's, but every Tuesday we had an adventure awaiting us beyond Short Creek. Early in the morning, we would load up in Papaw's two-seat Ford truck and hit the road to Hazard.

Once we arrived, Mamaw had me throwing elbows among men and women with twice my stature and a quarter of my patience—all for that one rare antique. Our grand destination was what we called the "Junk Store"; to this day, I still do not know the actual name of the store. Every Tuesday, we arrived there before the delivery trucks did so that we would be ready when the time came to snag the whatnot of our choice. There was one rule. You cannot grab an item until it has been placed on the shelf by the worker. A crowd gathered in anticipation around the double doors in the back of the store, and finally, a worker pushing a shopping cart full of antique knickknacks emerged. In that moment, Mamaw would tell me exactly what she wanted from the cart, and with the advantage of being a small child, I squeezed my way through the crowd until I was stalking the item of her choice, waiting for the store clerk to place it on the shelf like a salivating dog awaiting scraps under a table. As soon as the item touched the shelf, I would grab it. When she saw me emerge from the crowd with that special item, she was so tickled that she couldn't help but let out her shy, muffled giggle, hiding her smile behind her right hand. The Junk Store was always the highlight of our week. Once we returned home, we looked up the items we had just gotten in one of the three antique books that Mamaw had. She loved seeing how much they were worth, although she knew that she would keep them forever.

Once I started school, I saw that smile grow bigger and bigger when I came home every school year from the annual award ceremony with several class awards—all due to the investment she made in my education at an early age. When I was in fourth grade, my favorite part of the day was when I jumped off the bus to see Mamaw standing on the bridge, waiting for me to begin the seven-minute walk up the gravel driveway to her house. She smiled as I told her all about my school day, and she knew that every day she had a graded quiz awaiting her when we walked through the kitchen door. I quizzed her on everything I learned that day from the biology in Mrs. Nikki's class to the state symbols in Mrs. Crisp's class. She learned as much as I did that year and loved every minute of it.

When I was in middle school, I got a Nintendo Wii for Christmas, and of course, I took it to Mamaw and Papaw's. Papaw and I played the Wii for hours, and all three of us laughed so hard as Papaw tried several different stances and swings to perfect his golf game. Papaw and I played for hours, never growing tired of hearing the high-pitched "swoosh" sound that the remote made with every swing. Our Wii games were interrupted only by hot meals and checker matches. To wrap the night up, the three of us went to the kitchen table to play Rummy while we listened to the singing and preaching on WLJC-TV. Every turn, Papaw said, "Throw my card, Irene. Come on. Throw my card."

When I was a junior in high school, Mamaw was so happy to hear that I was going to be the valedictorian of my senior class, but that year, she was diagnosed with non–small-cell lung cancer. The doctor gave her until Christmas, but she fought for months after, remaining beautiful and golden through the chemo and radiation. It weakened her body but never her smile or childlike giggle. Mamaw wanted to live to see me walk down the aisle as valedictorian. She wanted to see me receive my medal and roses and give my speech. However, on a sunny day in early May, I was at softball practice with my friends when my phone was flooded with messages and missed calls. I left practice and drove thirty minutes to the Hospice Center. That day, Mamaw went on to Heaven—two weeks before I graduated with the highest honors due to the hours that she had spent with me as a young child—two weeks before the moment that she had been waiting to see for nineteen years. On graduation night, I honored her in my speech and dedicated my roses to her. I took them to her grave after the ceremony, and I thanked her for everything that she had done for me as I laid the roses on her grave. I hope that she liked those flowers as much as the ones we watered while holding hands together in the yard.

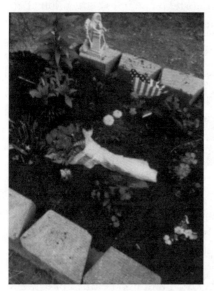

In sociology, I learned that health disparities are unjust and avoidable, and Appalachians are faced with many health disparities that include cancer, heart disease, diabetes, and more. It pains me to think that for so many Appalachians, if they had been born or lived somewhere else, they might still be alive. They might not have suffered. It is important for Appalachians to be aware of and acknowledge these differences in health due to location.

Southeastern Kentucky has always had health disparities dating back to the early 1900s when households were isolated. Due to the mountainous geography, travel and transportation was always a challenge in Leslie County. There were few roadways, and the few existing ones were hard to travel because they were unpaved. Because of the lack of roads, residents often traveled by horseback through creeks and on small trails across mountains. Many people lived deep in the mountains without access to electricity, phones, and indoor plumbing.

Due to the lack of education and social isolation of the mountains, Leslie County had a severe need for trained medical personnel. At the time, there was not a licensed doctor in Leslie County. Often, trained healthcare personnel did not want to move to Leslie County because the poverty of the area would make it almost impossible to collect monetary compensation. Occasionally, clinics were provided via outside sources, but most of the healthcare depended on traditional practices and remedies that were based only on experience and often superstition. This care often depended on "granny women," or women who provided care for others, particularly mothers and infants. Traditional healthcare practices such as prayer and folk-healing were free, while seeing a trained professional would cost money that the poverty-stricken residents of Leslie County could not spare. The closest trained medical professionals were in Hazard, which was over a day's ride away on horseback.[1] For every 100,000 children born, over 800 resulted in maternal death, while 100 out of 1,000 children did not live to see their first birthday.[2]

Although there has been substantial progress since the 1900s, some of these problems remain in Leslie County on a lesser scale. Many Leslie Countians travel over two hours to Lexington, Kentucky, to receive specialized medical treatment, whether it be to see a dermatologist, oncologist, endocrinologist, or other specialist. Many cannot afford or are simply not willing to travel so far. The cost and inconvenience of transportation is a contributing factor for Appalachians not getting the appropriate health screenings, leading to increased cancer rates.

When I went to Ecuador on a health brigade with the University of Kentucky Shoulder to Shoulder Global program, one of the most important things I learned in the training course and in my time in Ecuador is that in order to treat someone, you must understand his or her culture. Appalachia is full of beautiful, rich culture. Anyone who goes to Southeastern Kentucky leaves saying, "Those were some of the kindest people that I have ever met." We have deeply rooted traditions and customs in our diet, dialect, recreation, and social norms. To treat Appalachians, it is important to be knowledgeable about Appalachian culture.

Speaking from experience, I know it can be hard to gain the trust of Appalachians. When we speak in the mountains, we smile, make eye contact, and take our time. Because of our social norms, Appalachians often consider someone who is abrupt as rude, and unfortunately, it is also hard for Appalachians to trust those who do not meet our social norms. Our culture is so beautiful, but the mistrust that comes with it can also be harmful. For example, mistrust can lead to a fatalistic mindset. A fatalistic mindset is one in which one thinks his or her death is predetermined and that there is no use in fighting it. I often hear, "Well if I get cancer, then it is just my time to go." Instead of taking the time and spending the money to go get screenings or to get an ominous symptom checked, too many Appalachians fall back on this fatalistic mantra. Lack of trust also causes many Appalachians to not trust doctors, whether the doctors are in Lexington or Hyden. They often think that doctors are simply trying to make money off of them by having them run tests or by having them follow up. Because of the mistrust, individuals often do not adhere to the plan of treatment suggested by their healthcare providers.

As it did in the early 1900s, the economy also still plays a large role in health disparities in Appalachia. Southeastern Kentucky is notably one of the poorest regions in the nation. In many Appalachian towns, there is not a whole lot to do aside from enjoying the gorgeous scenery. There are not many jobs, and as the saying goes, idle hands do the devil's work. Because of the poor economy, lack of jobs, and lack of recreation, depression can take over. Some turn to recreational drugs and excessive drinking to cope. When under the influence of drugs or alcohol, individuals partake in riskier behaviors such as smoking or sexual activities—both of which increase risk of cancer. Because of the economy, people also cannot afford to go to the doctor if they have symptoms such as a persistently bad cough or a mole that has irregular borders. They often wait until their symptoms are unbearable because they simply cannot afford the bills that come with the visit.

Another cultural factor is the "Man Box." I learned in sociology that the Man Box is the social construction of what a man should or should not be. In Southeastern Kentucky, the Man Box is very much an issue. Most Appalachians—particularly men and boys—are taught that if you go to the doctor, then you are weak. You have to "tough it out," or you will be teased and labeled as "not man enough." This often leads to later detection of cancer and a worse prognosis.

My goal is to research and study Appalachian health disparities as an oncologist and to return home to treat Appalachians. In order for the health disparities in Appalachia to improve, we need more Appalachians involved in Appalachian healthcare. As in the early 1900s, there are not many who want to move to Southeastern Kentucky. One reason is that they are not rooted here. Second, the economy is not great, and there is not a whole lot that attracts newcomers other than the beautiful environment. We need Leslie Countians to help Leslie County.

Increased health education can also improve cancer outcomes in Appalachia. The health literacy in Appalachia needs to be improved greatly. Basic medical terminology should be taught in school curriculum in addition to skills to improve health literacy. These skills include taking notes while in the doctor's office and coming to the visit prepared with a list of symptoms and questions. Health literacy skills should be pushed in all schools but especially in areas such as Appalachia where the health disparities are so great.

My role model is the woman for which the hospital I was born in was named: Mary Carson Breckinridge. In the 1900s, she improved the infant mortality rates in Leslie County greatly by riding on horseback from house to house to provide care and by establishing the Frontier Nursing University, multiple clinics, and a hospital. Through forty years of service,

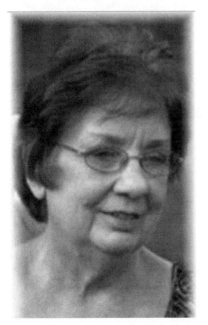

57,640 patients were registered in her clinic. Babies and toddlers accounted for 24,809 of these patients, along with 9,698 school children and 23,133 adults. There were 27,903 patients admitted to Hyden Hospital, and most impressively, there were only eleven maternal deaths in those forty years.[3] Following the path of Mary Breckinridge, I would like to return home and ease the cancer burden in Leslie County by improving health literacy, by creating outreach programs, and by treating each patient as I would have treated my own grandmother.

In Loving Memory of Irene Brock

Notes

1. Melanie Goans, "'First, Foremost, and Above All for Babies': Mary Breckinridge and the Frontier Nursing Service," 2000, University of Kentucky, 56–340.

2. https://www.cdc.gov/mmwr/preview/mmwrhtml/mm4838a2.htm.

3. Katherine Wilkie and Elizabeth Moseley, "Frontier Nurse: Mary Breckinridge," *Messner,* 1969, 184.

Malignancy in the Mountains

Susanna Goggans

GENERATIONS OF MY mom's family are buried in a tiny graveyard on top of a hill in Red Bush, Kentucky. Although many of my relatives moved away through the years, my grandparents and other family members remain in Red Bush. Even though I grew up in the next town over, Paintsville, I will always consider Red Bush my home. All our family celebrations and reunions are in Red Bush. Growing up in Eastern Kentucky, I learned how to fish, hike, and make cornbread, but most importantly, I learned the value of loyalty. Eastern Kentuckians are loyal to one another, to their friends, to their neighbors, and, most of all, to family. There is a sense of community in which everyone looks out for one another, whether it is giving a neighbor some homegrown tomatoes or helping rebuild houses when Red Bush was flooded. When I realized the true value of this support, however, was when my mom was diagnosed with ovarian cancer.

Once a year, my mom and my grandma would drive to Prestonsburg to get a free screening from the University of Kentucky's (UK) Ovarian Cancer Screening Program. My grandma had heard about it through her local homemaker's group she attends once a week, and my mom and grandma would always make a day of it, doing some local shopping and going out to eat after their screening. It was my mom's fourth time getting screened when a cyst was discovered, so they made an appointment at UK a few weeks later. They told her she should get her ovary removed, and my mom opted to have a total hysterectomy. The surgery was scheduled for May 23. I was a freshman at UK at the time, and I was home for the summer that first week of May. I found the fact that she had to get surgery, frankly, annoying. Her CA 125, a blood test that serves as a tumor marker, was barely elevated, and while they knew she had a cyst on her ovary, nobody seemed concerned that it would actually be cancer. I thought they were just being extra-precautionary, and I had no reason to worry. May 23 came around, and I was at home taking care of my sister, who has severe cerebral palsy, while my dad took my mom to UK for surgery.

The surgery was supposed to last two hours. I am a pre-med student, and I had observed a hysterectomy before, and I knew that my mom's surgery would be through the da Vinci robot and, therefore, be minimally invasive, so there shouldn't be complications. However, my mom went into surgery very early that morning, and time kept ticking. I took my sister to school at 8:00 a.m.; I went to my local hospital to get an observer's badge at 11:00 a.m.; I went to get lunch at 12:00 p.m., and I knew the surgery shouldn't still be going on. I kept texting my dad, and he assured me the doctors said she was doing fine. I kept telling myself, "Maybe she's out and he just forgot to tell me. I am sure it is hectic." But time just kept ticking. At 2:00 p.m., I got a phone call from my dad. The second I saw the phone ringing, my heart sank. I know my dad, and I knew he'd just text me to say, "She's out," if all was okay. I knew the surgery had lasted way too long. He said, "Well, it is both the best news and the worst news. They found cancer, but it was deep inside her ovary. The doctor thinks it hasn't spread. They've spent the last four hours taking samples from different areas, making sure the cancer hasn't spread."

It was diagnosed to be ovarian cancer stage 1a, grade 3. It was found as early as possible, still contained inside her ovary. However, it was the highest grade, meaning she needed to go through six rounds of chemotherapy just in case one sneaky cancer cell escaped. Ovarian cancer is called the silent killer because there are often no symptoms until stage 3 or 4, often too late. I knew that my mom was extremely lucky to get to have an end date on her chemotherapy treatments, and I used the thought that she would eventually be okay in order to stay positive and optimistic through her treatments. That summer, I was the "mom" of the family, taking care of my sister while my mom was recovering from surgery and too exhausted from her chemotherapy treatments.

The chemotherapy treatments started mid-June. They were every three weeks, and Lexington is a two-hour drive from Paintsville. Going to Lexington and back in one day is exhausting for anyone, even if they're not receiving a three-hour treatment of poison in their veins. I could tell that both my mom and dad, who took her to that treatment, were completely drained by the time they arrived back home that evening. The first treatment wasn't too bad. My mom felt almost normal, just a little tired, and she didn't start losing her hair until almost the next treatment. I volunteered to drive her to the next two appointments, as I knew I would be returning to school soon and would not have the chance to give my dad a break from the drive then. These appointments were, honestly, fun. We called them "chemo parties," and my mom's first cousin, her daughter, and my mom's friend would come visit. We all laughed and talked the entire time, probably greatly disturbing the peace of the Markey Cancer Center. However, it made time pass, and it seemed to make my mom forget what she was there for.

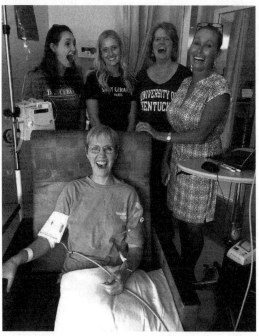

Four more chemo parties after this one, and my mom was finished with treatment! The support that came from family and our community was phenomenal. Everywhere I went, I had people asking me how she was doing and sending their prayers. She got many cards in the mail and many comments on Facebook posts; people seemed to be offering their help left and right. The women in my family all made Ovarian Cancer Awareness shirts to wear and are now all very strong advocates of the Ovarian Cancer Screening Program.

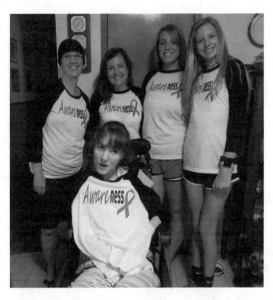

I will always be thankful for the support my family felt during these difficult times. That summer, I was curious about how my seemingly healthy mom who exercised almost every day and ate mostly nutritious, home-cooked food could ever have a tumor growing inside of her. I still do not exactly know that answer, but I did learn that Kentucky, especially Eastern Kentucky, is plagued with terrifyingly high cancer rates. While ovarian cancer is not one that is particularly high in Eastern Kentucky, lung, colorectal, and cervical cancers have taken over this region.[1] I believe this is due to limited access to healthcare and high rates of obesity and smoking, with poverty worsening each of these factors.[2] All of these are related to create the perfect storm for cancer to take root.

As I mentioned while telling my mom's cancer story, doctors are far away, especially specialists. For people living in the rural areas of my county, it can take thirty or forty minutes to drive into town (Paintsville) just to get a checkup. This makes getting the recommended screenings a much larger burden. Without early detection, cancer can progress to a later stage, making it more difficult to treat. Additionally, if something is found, as in the case of my mom, and the patient is recommended to see a specialist, the drive to Lexington is over three hours for those on the farthest end of

Eastern Kentucky. For those who are struggling financially, this drive could be almost impossible, or at least more trouble than it seems worth to the patient. This could lead to the patient's not following up and thus allowing their cancer to advance.

The lifestyle in Eastern Kentucky also contributes to the cancer rates, and the two elements that I believe contribute most to cancer are obesity and smoking. Being overweight or obese is associated with an increased risk of cancer, and Eastern Kentucky has limited access to exercise facilities, a culturally unhealthy diet, and high levels of poverty, all of which contribute to the high obesity rates.[3] For the people that live out in the country, it can be difficult to find the time and motivation to drive into town to go to a tiny gym. On top of that, the classic Eastern Kentucky foods I grew up eating at my grandma's, such as fried okra, cornbread, and fried chicken, do not promote a healthy diet (while they are delicious). Poverty leads to less money to buy more expensive fresh fruits and vegetables and makes it easier to opt for cheaper, processed fast food. The culture doesn't promote eating healthy and exercising, and that is contributing to more obesity and more cancer.

Smoking is the most frustrating factor in Eastern Kentucky, in my opinion. It has been well known for decades that smoking leads to lung cancer, yet people still smoke. I do not know exactly why people decide to start an addictive behavior they know is so detrimental to their health, but this has led to Kentucky having the highest rates of lung cancer in the nation.[4] Smoking is more common in populations with higher poverty and lower education rates, both of which have contributed to Eastern Kentucky's addiction to cigarettes. Hopefully, eventually smoking will go out of style.

Decreasing the cancer rate in Eastern Kentucky is not a simple task due to the variety of factors contributing to the cancer rates in complex ways. However, awareness, I believe, will make the biggest difference. In 2000, the Kentucky Cancer Consortium began an awareness campaign to help improve colorectal screenings, and this has led to a 25 percent drop in the incidence of colorectal cancer.[5] This is a major improvement, and it shows how effective awareness campaigns can be.

We should start increasing awareness by teaching kids in schools more about cancer. We can educate them about necessary screenings and healthy lifestyle choices in order to decrease their chances of getting cancer. This would instill the message in kids while they are young so that, hopefully, they would be more likely to take the preventative efforts that decrease their risk for cancer as they grow older. In the meantime, educational materials should be spread to communities through posts on Facebook, speakers at churches, and any other place the community gathers in order to educate the public about the importance of staying up to date with their screenings and living a healthy lifestyle. After my mom shared her story on Facebook, she got many messages from people telling her they were going to get screened for ovarian cancer. Spreading the message makes a difference. It may not be dramatic at first, but slowly it can decrease Kentucky's cancer mortality rate.

If I learned anything from last summer, it was to always stay positive. Even though watching my mom go through chemo was difficult, I watched her power through and keep going, strongly trenching through the cancer path to the finish line. Cancer is a devastating disease, and while we do not yet have the cure, we are not powerless. We can fight it by catching it before it advances or preventing it from ever forming. Eastern Kentucky is behind in the fight, but I am confident we will eventually catch up. I am positive that Eastern Kentucky, with some help, will be able to fight through the cancer epidemic and become a healthier place.

Notes

1. American Cancer Society, "Cancer Facts & Statistics—Kentucky," 2019, retrieved June 26, 2019, from https://cancerstatisticscenter.cancer.org/#!/state/Kentucky.

2. B. Estep, "Death Comes Sooner in Appalachia. It Comes Much Sooner in Eastern Kentucky," August 24, 2017, retrieved from https://www.kentucky.com/news/state/article169037857.html.

3. S. Zuppello, "The Cancer Capital of America," May 22, 2019, retrieved from https://theoutline.com/post/7457/the-cancer-capital-of-america?zd=2&zi=dfaangls.

4. American Lung Association, "Kentucky Lung Cancer Rates," February 27, 2018, retrieved from https://www.lung.org/our-initiatives/research/monitoring-trends-in-lung-disease/state-of-lung-cancer/states/KY.html.

5. Zuppello, "Cancer Capital."

A Rural State of Mind on the Path to a Better Future

Matthew Melton

MY NAME IS Matthew Melton. I am from a small area of Eastern Kentucky called Powell County. Kentucky is known for many things, including bourbon, horse racing, the beautiful, rolling hills of the Appalachian Mountains, and many other wonders. Although there are many reasons to love Kentucky, there are hidden concerns.

Growing up in Powell County, I knew that health disparities were very prominent in daily life. From heart health, to diabetes, to cancers, it seemed that my peers and our families were doomed for bad health. I can distinctly recall attending funerals for family and friends who had passed away from diseases that are far too common in Kentucky: lung cancers, breast cancers, strokes, and more. Despite the impending doom that seemed to be present in my future, coupled with the economic difficulties of my family and Eastern Kentucky, I knew I wanted to help others.

Based on the history that I have, I decided to seek a career in the medical field as a family physician, first by attaining a public health bachelor's degree at the University of Kentucky and then by attending medical school.

Beyond family and friend interactions, my own personal experiences with cancer did not begin until high school, when I was in a dual-credit chemistry class. During this class, we took a field trip to test natural waters around Powell County for carcinogens. After testing the waters, we found heavy metals, fertilizers, and other dangerous chemicals. Finding chemicals in the water was a huge concern and resulted in having the class attend a conference about cancers in the area. The conference was led by researchers in charge of the chemical weapons depot in Richmond, Kentucky.

This sparked my interests in cancer and resulted in submitting my application for a position in a new program started by the Markey Cancer Center for Appalachian students seeking a career in oncology. Upon my acceptance, I was flung into the world of medicine, and I could not have been more excited. Over the next three years, I would watch a vast number of oncological surgeries, shadow in cancer clinics, and complete my own research in cancer therapeutics. This is where my personality and desires truly flourished. All my life I had wanted to be a part of the medical world, and the experiences that I was able to gain from shadowing oncologists were more than I had ever dreamed of. To name a few, I was able to see a total laryngectomy and several hysterectomies and to participate in conversations with world-renowned researchers at the 2019 American Association for Cancer Research annual meeting.

Now, as a senior in college, I have applied and been accepted to attend medical school, and I feel that I have gained a wealth of knowledge in cancer treatments and future prevention. From diet to UV light exposure to carcinogens in our communities, I believe that the future of cancer treatment will lie in prevention. Due to the vast number of cancers and cancer subtypes, a vaccine or cure-all drug will likely never be created. Instead, the best treatment for cancer will be preventing the occurrence at all.

Kentucky is a hotspot for cancers, ranking as the worst state for cancer deaths. Cancer is the second leading cause of death in the state, with over ten thousand deaths, behind heart disease.[1] I would assume that there are a variety of factors that create these astounding rates, but I also believe it is likely heavily tied to chemicals that we ingest on a daily basis in our water. Kentucky's tap waters have been tested and repeatedly found to contain toxic heavy metals, benzene, chlorine, fluoride, arsenic, lead, dimethyl disulfide, carbon disulfide, naphthalene, trimethyl benzene, and many other dangerous chemicals.[2] If Kentucky hopes to decrease the rates of cancers, I believe that it is very important to decrease the levels of cancer-causing chemicals and metals in the tap water. Additionally, the diets in Kentucky are comprised of abnormally high amounts of fatty meats. Fatty meats have been linked to several types of cancers, and healthier diets could be a preventative factor to certain types of cancers.[3] Perhaps educational or legislative changes should be made to encourage healthier eating in Kentucky, similar to changes that have been made by the U.S. Department of Agriculture in public school systems.[4]

Overall, Kentucky is a beautiful state, with a variety of unique wonders and people. However, there are also many health concerns that Kentucky citizens face. Now, Kentucky and the world must fight for all of our futures. We must challenge ourselves to become healthier and create a world that is free of cancer-causing chemicals.

Notes

1. Centers for Disease Control and Prevention, "Stats of the States—Cancer Mortality," 2019, retrieved June 18, 2019, from https://www.cdc.gov/nchs/pressroom/sosmap/cancer_mortality/cancer.htm.

2. Apec Health, "Carcinogenic Chemicals in the Water Supply: Is Your Tap Water Safe?" 2018, retrieved June 18, 2019, from https://www.freedrinkingwater.com/water_health/cancer-tap-water-contaminants-link.htm.

3. Department of Health and Human Services, "Cancer and Food," March 31, 2014, retrieved June 18, 2019, from https://www.betterhealth.vic.gov.au/health/conditionsand treatments/cancer-and-food.

4. USDA-FNS, "USDA Proposes Standards to Provide Healthy Food Options in Schools," 2013, retrieved June 18, 2019, from https://www.fns.usda.gov/pressrelease /2013/001913.

Fighting Cancer in My Old Kentucky Home

Carrigan Wasilchenko

AS I'M DRIVING down the narrow road I grew up on, it seems as if nothing has changed. The trees, the landscape, and the livestock all appear the same as they were when I was a child many years ago. The smell of the air is even the same: a little musty with a hint of pine. I pull into my old driveway and make my way to the porch swing. The house is empty now, but I can almost believe that my mother is just inside about to prepare dinner. I become nostalgic when I realize how everything has stayed the same as I have grown tremendously. I begin to think about my life, where I came from and how far I have come, and I am overcome with emotion.

For the entirety of my life, I have felt a deep connection to the rolling hills of Kentucky. I love the culture, the location, and most of all, I love the people. The people of Kentucky are those who adopted me as their own, even though I was born in another country. Kentuckians taught me the importance of family, tradition, and determination. Most importantly, my beloved fellow Kentuckians inspired me to become a physician.

My name is Carrigan Wasilchenko, and I grew up in Stanton, Kentucky. When I was a child growing up in Eastern Kentucky, Loretta Lynn, Ale 8, and quilting were all staples in my household. On any given day, I could expect to come home from school with a full homecooked meal on the table, followed by the matriarchs of the family gathering together in the living room to quilt. As they progressed, they would reflect on old memories and sing songs such as Loretta Lynn's "Blue Kentucky Girl." These seemingly mundane experiences are actually the ones I remember the most vividly, as they truly encapsulate the heart of Appalachia. Over the years, I received numerous quilts from my great-aunt and grandmother. Every time I use a quilt they made for me, I am reminded of the love that was sewn into every stitch and am comforted that they live on through some of the best traditions of Appalachia.

While I have experienced the best of Appalachian culture, I have also experienced the socioeconomic struggles that many of my fellow Kentuckians face. The town in Eastern Kentucky where I grew up struggles with unemployment, low incomes, the inability to attain higher education, low access to healthcare, and lower life expectancies. Due to these socioeconomic stressors, Kentuckians experience some of the worst health outcomes in America. Kentuckians experience higher rates of diabetes, heart disease, obesity, and even cancer when compared to the national average.[1] Although all of the aforementioned diseases can be fatal, cancer evokes the most heart-wrenching emotions, and for good reason.

Cancer is a disease that has ravaged Eastern Kentucky for as long as I can remember. Whether it be lung, breast, or even colon cancer, one thing is for certain: it discriminates against no one. Cancer knows no age, no gender, and it certainly doesn't know how much you love a person diagnosed with it. One of my earliest memories is going to visit my grandmother in the hospital. Although I was only seven years old, I can still remember the smell of the hospital, the visitors in the hallways, and the doctors in their white coats moving from room to room to care for their patients. My grandmother had just had surgery to remove a malignant tumor, but of course I didn't know that at the time. I can remember the surgeon regretfully shaking his head, telling my family that they were unable to fully resect it. He went on to explain other treatments that my grandmother would be eligible for. We followed his recommendations, but unfortunately, they were not enough. My grandmother passed away less than a year later. As a young child, I had difficulty in coping with the grief of losing a loved one, especially to a disease I didn't understand. In the years following my grandmother's death, more members of my family were diagnosed with varying forms of cancer, including my mother. I wish I could say the cases and emotions I've experienced in my own family were unique, but they were not.

My personal experiences with this disease inspired me to delve into the research that has been conducted in Kentucky. The data I found was startling—on average, Kentuckians experience some of the highest rates of lung, breast, colorectal, and cervical cancers in the nation.[2] In addition, the statistics worsen the farther into Appalachia you travel. According to the National Cancer Institute's (NCI) Incidence Rates Table, my hometown of Powell County has the highest incidence rate of cancer in Kentucky when selected for all cancer sites, all races, all sexes, and all ages.[3]

Prompted by my interest in and concern for the cancer epidemic of Kentucky, I applied for the Appalachian Career Training in Oncology (ACTION) Program. With the ACTION program, I have had the opportunity to observe surgeries, shadow oncologists, conduct cancer-focused research, and participate in community outreach. While shadowing at the University of Kentucky (UK) Markey Cancer Center, I observed the direct impact of socioeconomic and geographic disparities on cancer patients. Many of the patients treated at the Markey Cancer Center experience transportation barriers and immense financial hardships. For example, a few months ago, I spoke with a patient who told me that they were afraid of not being able to continue their chemotherapy treatments. When asked why they were afraid, the patient told me it was very difficult to find transportation to Lexington from their home two hours away. In another instance, I witnessed a phone call in which a patient was informed that their insurance would not cover their treatment, and that their current medical bill stood at more than $400,000. Eye-opening experiences such as these have enabled me to envision my goals for the future.

I dream of a world where no one ever has to hear the words "You have cancer." However, as a realist, I understand that this world is many years away, but there are still things that we can do to help decrease the cancer burden in Kentucky. First and foremost, we as Kentuckians must work together to advocate for and implement lifestyle changes—starting with smoking cessation. According to the *Northern Kentucky Tribune,* more Kentuckians have died from lung cancer than all of the other seven leading cancers combined.[4] Additionally, Kentucky suffers from high obesity rates, poor nutrition, and the consumption of potentially hazardous material in our water supply due to coal mining. Many Kentuckians do not realize that these unhealthy behaviors can actually increase their risk of developing cancer. In addition to partaking in unhealthy behaviors, many Kentuckians do not undergo regular cancer screening. According to the Centers for Disease Control and Prevention, it is estimated that only 65.5 percent of age-eligible Kentucky residents had undergone colorectal cancer screening in 2012.[5] This statistic has improved in the years since, but the geographic disparities in Eastern Kentucky are still apparent. For many of the eastern counties, the use of a colorectal cancer screening test lies between 40.1–61.2 percent or 61.3–64.2 percent.[6] It is of the utmost importance that we begin assiduously educating Kentuckians about the importance of a healthy lifestyle, smoking cessation, and cancer screening.

However, it is not enough to educate Kentuckians on what behaviors to partake in and which ones to avoid. Kentuckians deserve better access to high-quality and reliable cancer care. Of all the cancer centers in the state, only one is designated by the National Cancer Institute (NCI). This designation means that a facility possesses strong scientific leadership, numerous resources, and a drive to develop cutting-edge approaches to prevent, diagnose, and treat cancer. There is a reason that people from all over the state come to the UK Markey Cancer Center for care. There is a reason that they bypass treatment facilities closer to home. Patients want the best care possible, so they make the long trek to Lexington in order to receive it.

Although having an NCI Designated Cancer Center is something to be proud of, I believe it is also something that we need to expand on. According to the CDC, Kentucky is ranked #1 in cancer mortality rates, yet we have only one NCI Designated Cancer Center.[7] California, on the other hand, is ranked #45 in cancer mortality rates and has eight Comprehensive Cancer Centers, which are even more advanced than Designated Cancer Centers.[8] It is not only necessary but logical for Kentucky to be home to more than one NCI Designated Cancer Center. The state of Kentucky needs to place an emphasis on funding for the development of more advanced facilities throughout the commonwealth. Kentuckians deserve the best care possible, and the best care is impossible to give when patients must travel unreasonably long distances to receive it.

I aspire to become an oncologist so I may one day be in a position to improve health outcomes and patient satisfaction for all Kentuckians. Ultimately, I hope to advocate for the construction of a specialized cancer treatment center in my hometown and other underserved rural areas. The people of Kentucky would benefit greatly from the establishment of specialized cancer facilities in these areas. It would allow patients to obtain treatment closer to home accompanied by friends and family, eliminate barriers to essential preventive screenings, and provide excellent opportunities for coordinating cancer awareness/prevention campaigns across the Bluegrass State. In order to ameliorate the issues in our great commonwealth, we as healthcare professionals must provide the resources to treat, educate, and advocate for the improvement of health so that our unbridled spirit may reign on.

Eastern Kentucky is the place that I've called home for the past twenty years. I will never grow tired of the rolling hills, the thick accents, or the ever-present availability of Ale 8. My experiences in this amazing state will continue to be the driving force behind my determination and will to fight for the care that all Kentuckians deserve. One day I hope to become a physician who can help change the health landscape of the Bluegrass, a place I'm so proud to call home, for the better.

Notes

1. United Health Foundation, "America's Health Rankings: Analysis of America's Health Rankings Composite Measure," 2018, retrieved from https://www.americashealthrankings.org/explore/annual/measure/Overall/state/KY.

2. National Cancer Institute, "State Cancer Profiles: Quick Profiles Kentucky," 2019, retrieved from https://statecancerprofiles.cancer.gov/quick-profiles/index.php?statename=kentucky.

3. National Cancer Institute, "State Cancer Profiles: Incidence Rates Table," 2019, retrieved from https://statecancerprofiles.cancer.gov/incidencerates/index.php?stateFIPS=21&cancer=001&race=00&sex=0&age=001&type=incd&sortVariableName=rate&sortOrder=default#results.

4. *Northern Kentucky Tribune*, "KY has high rates of lung cancer and high rates of smoking; lung cancer can be prevented and treated," 2017, https://www.nkytribune.com/2017/11/ky-has-high-rates-of-lung-cancer-and-high-rates-of-smoking-lung-cancer-can-be-prevented-and-treated/.

5. Centers for Disease Control and Prevention, "Quick Facts: Colorectal Screening Test Use in Kentucky Behavioral Risk Factor Surveillance System 2016," 2016, retrieved from https://www.cdc.gov/cancer/ncccp/screening-rates/pdf/colorectal-cancer-screening-kentucky-508.pdf.

6. Ibid.

7. Centers for Disease Control and Prevention, "Cancer Mortality by State," 2019, retrieved from https://www.cdc.gov/nchs/pressroom/sosmap/cancer_mortality/cancer.htm.

8. National Cancer Institute, "Find a Cancer Center," 2019, retrieved from https://www.cancer.gov/research/nci-role/cancer-centers/find.

Roots

Emory Wilds

I am from sunshine,
From soil and summer nights.
I am from the creek across the field,
Rushing, wild, and free.
I am from the moon, the woods
Whose arms welcomed me
As if they were my home.

I am from chicken and blackberries,
From squash blooms and biscuits.
I am from the sounds of life,
Howling wolves and croaking frogs.
I am from the sweet air, the spring rain
With muddy feet
And a mind that never stops wandering.

I am from dirt roads and honeysuckles,
From fireflies in a mason jar.
I am from the yard with a willow tree,
Blowing freely in the wind.
I am from the backbreaking work in the garden,
With sweat trickling down my neck,
A warm summer breeze dancing across my skin.

I am from these moments.
A warrior from the wildflowers.

> Though I have roots,
> They do not hold down my feet.

I AM FROM Eastern Kentucky. This statement alone will often cause me to be undeservedly stereotyped, but the complexities of one's cultural identity cannot be summed up by preconceived notions. Growing up in rural Kentucky gave me an appreciation for the importance of nature, an understanding of the necessity of hard work, and the ability to embody the contradictory values of both stability from deep family roots and fierce independence from ingrained self-determination. At the same time, I have seen the damaging impact of economic, environmental, and educational barriers on the health and well-being of those living around me. The negative effects of these barriers are reflected in my community through high rates of cancer, opioid addiction, and mental illness—all made worse by poor education and a lack of access to medical care.

Since coming to the University of Kentucky (UK), my involvement in the Markey Cancer Center Appalachian Career Training in Oncology (ACTION) Program has provided me with incredible opportunities that have developed my understanding of the health issues so prevalent in Eastern Kentucky. One of my first moments of realization was learning about the connections between social determinants such as income, education level, social support, environment, and resource access on one's life expectancy and ability to remain healthy. I came to understand that structural inequalities and social determinants can be found within any defined group of people regardless of race, place, creed, or identity. These determinants are primary contributing factors to the reality that the nation's highest cancer prevalence and death rates are found in Eastern Kentucky.[1]

In my own family, I had a grandpa pass from lung cancer, another with prostate cancer. I have a grandmother with thyroid cancer, the other with skin cancer. Although cancer seemingly "runs in my family," the reality is that my grandparents' shared environment, resource accessibility, and lifestyle choices—such as tobacco use and unprotected sun exposure—most likely had more impact on their health than inherited genes. Part of the battle toward better health outcomes is simply being aware of the barriers that exist for individuals like my grandparents and having the willingness to find ways to address them. Through the ACTION Program, I have experienced the power of local outreach in educating people about prevention, community resources, and the importance of early life-saving cancer screening.

Another moment of clarity came through an ACTION clinical observation experience at the UK Markey Cancer Center with a surgical gynecologic oncologist. Although my initial goal was to explore oncology in general, this particular experience focusing on women's health issues had a great impact on me. Beyond the burden of a cancer diagnosis, which is difficult for any person, gynecological oncology issues add another layer of incredibly intimate and personal decision-making that can affect a person's identity as a woman as well as her future reproductive health. Imagine making the decision to undergo a surgery that could result in never being able to start a family in the traditional way we all take for granted. These kinds of decisions were part of developing treatment plans, revealing how complex these situations can be. The use of a variety of different specialties and related support services—everything from reconstructive surgery to oncofertility to mental health services to integrative therapies—showed me the importance of a holistic and personalized approach to medicine. Because of my rural background, I believe in the connection between the mind, body, and environment, and I was able to see and understand the value of holistically addressing a person's needs during my time in this observation rotation.

These experiences have been pivotal points for me, opening my eyes to the complexities of cancer and inspiring an interest in a future in oncology. I have gained new perspectives about the extreme healthcare needs in my own home area, which can be addressed only through comprehensive prevention and treatment efforts. I continue to have unexpected moments of learning with every experience in this field and envision that the medical profession is a lifelong process of discovery. Through community outreach efforts, I am learning we must keep our humility in check in order to educate without belittling. After observing physicians guiding patients through difficult life decisions, I am seeing that we must respect patient autonomy without patronizing. In order to achieve the most successful and lasting health outcomes, we must understand the value of engaging support services for patients without making them feel inept. William Osler said, "The good physician treats the disease; the great physician treats the patient who has the disease." I have been privileged to learn from health professionals and mentors at UK who are exemplifying Osler's words by working together toward lessening the cancer burden for those who, like myself and my grandparents, call Eastern Kentucky home.

Notes

1. National Cancer Institute, "SEER Cancer Statistics Review (CSR), 1975–2016," 2019, retrieved from https://seer.cancer.gov/csr/1975_2016/sections.html.

Acknowledgments

Funding for this project was provided by the University of Kentucky (UK) Office for Institutional Diversity, the UK Chellgren Center, and the Markey Cancer Foundation. Special thanks go to Dr. Sonja Feist-Price (Vice President for Institutional Diversity), Dr. Philipp Kraemer (Director of the Chellgren Center), and Michael Delzotti (President and CEO of the Markey Cancer Foundation). Thank you all for your support and trust!

The Appalachian Career Training in Oncology (ACTION) Program is funded by the National Cancer Institute (NCI R25CA221765).

Thank you to the University Press of Kentucky for publishing these essays as this book. I really appreciate the Press's enthusiasm for and dedication to ensuring the quality of the project.

Thank you to all the students who worked extraordinarily hard on writing these essays! You all did such a great job! Great work. I am very proud of all of you.

I owe much to Lauren Hudson and Chris Prichard who worked diligently with me in editing the essays and keeping the students on task! Thank you!

Thanks to the Markey Cancer Center's administrative staff in the director's office and in the center's Research Communications Office for administrative support.

Very special thanks to all the parents, guardians, and extended family for trusting us with your children and in your strong support of the mission of the ACTION Program. Without your support and trust, we would not be able to accomplish our goals. Thank you!

Nathan L. Vanderford, PhD, MBA
Director, Appalachian Career Training
in Oncology (ACTION) Program

About the Editors

Nathan L. Vanderford was born and raised in the small, southern-middle Tennessee town of Leoma (Lawrence County) that is in the Appalachian region.

He earned both a Bachelor of Science degree in Agricultural Biotechnology in 1999 and a Doctor of Philosophy degree in Biochemistry in 2008 from the University of Kentucky (UK). He also completed a Master of Business Administration degree from Midway University in 2013.

He is an assistant professor at the UK College of Medicine within the Department of Toxicology and Cancer Biology. He also holds several administrative positions including Assistant Director for Research for the Markey Cancer Center, Director of Administration for the Center for Cancer and Metabolism, and Director of the Appalachian Career Training in Oncology Program at UK. In these administrative positions, he works to facilitate research and education initiatives across the university.

Nathan has an award-winning history of teaching and mentoring students and in creating innovative career-development experiences and opportunities for students, including designing and directing the ACTION Program. He is the author of over fifty articles appearing in scientific journals and is co-author of a book titled *ReSearch: A Career Guide for Scientists*. His work has been covered in leading scientific journals (for example, *Nature* and *Science*) and by the popular press, including *Inside Higher Ed, U.S. News and World Report*, and *The Atlantic*.

Nathan lives in Lexington, Kentucky, with his wife and two children. He can be reached through his website: www.nathanvanderford.com. He can be found on Twitter @nlvanderford.

Lauren Hudson is a native of Villa Hills, Kentucky (Kenton County). She graduated from Dixie Heights High School in 2018 and is currently pursuing a Bachelor's in Neuroscience and Biology with a minor in Spanish at the University of Kentucky (UK). She plans to attend medical school following undergraduate graduation in 2022.

At the University of Kentucky, Lauren is the parliamentarian for a national co-ed service fraternity, Alpha Phi Omega. She is also a member of the UK club soccer team and is heavily involved in cancer research with the Markey Cancer Center. In the summer of 2019, she was a resident advisor for the Appalachian Career Training in Oncology Program residential summer program.

In addition to her passion for medicine, Lauren is an award-winning author of two book series. First, she began co-authoring the *Students Leading America* series with her father in 2013. In 2016, she released her first novel in the *Ascension* series, a young-adult fantasy trilogy, with the sequel following in 2018. Lauren has won awards worldwide and has traveled to London, New York, Cincinnati, and Los Angeles to speak. She also adapted the first book in the *Ascension* series into a screenplay, which won in over half a dozen film festivals across the nation.

Chris Prichard was raised in Frenchburg, Kentucky (Menifee County), in the heart of Kentucky's Appalachian region. He earned a Bachelor of Arts degree in English and Secondary Education in 2008 from Morehead State University. He is currently pursuing a Master of Higher Education degree from the University of Kentucky.

Chris has worked with secondary students throughout Eastern Kentucky for over ten years. He worked with the Upward Bound Programs at Morehead State University from 2012 to 2018. He is currently the program coordinator for the Appalachian Career Training in Oncology Program at the University of Kentucky's Markey Cancer Center.